Health Matters!

Volume 1
Addiction: Tobacco, Alcohol, and Other Drugs

General Editor

William M. Kane, Ph.D.
University of New Mexico

Advisors

Marilee Foglesong
Former Young Adult Coordinator
New York Public Library

James Robinson III, Ed.D.
Texas A&M University

Stephen Stewart, DrPH
James Madison University

GROLIER

Old Sherman Turnpike
Danbury, Connecticut 06816

Published 2002 by Grolier Educational
Old Sherman Turnpike
Danbury, CT 06816

Developed, Designed, and Produced by BOOK BUILDERS LLC

Set ISBN: 0-7172-5575-1
Vol. 1 ISBN: 0-7172-5576-X

For information address the publisher:
Grolier Educational, Old Sherman Turnpike, Danbury, CT 06816

Photo Credits
The following photographs are used by permission and through the courtesy of CMSP: 6, 29, 60, 68, 81 (J. Meyer), 101 (SPL), 106 (A. Wilson), 109, 120, and 155 (J. Meyer).

Every endeavor has been made to obtain permission to use copyrighted material.
The publishers would appreciate errors or omissions being brought to their attention.

Library of Congress Cataloging-in-Publication Data

Health matters!
        p. cm.
        Contents: v. 1. Addiction: tobacco, alcohol, and other drugs—v. 2. Mental health depression, suicide, and other issues—v. 3. Sexuality and pregnancy—v. 4. Physical activity, weight, and eating disorders—v. 5. Injuries and violence—v. 6. Environmental poisoning—v. 7. HIV infections, AIDS, and STDs—v. 8. Diseases and disabling conditions.
        ISBN 0-7172-5575-1 (set: alk. paper)—ISBN 0-7172-5576-X (v. 1: alk. paper)—
ISBN 0-7172-5577-8 (v. 2: alk. paper)—ISBN 0-7172-5578-6 (v. 3: alk. paper)—
ISBN 0-7172-5579-4 (v. 4: alk. paper)—ISBN 0-7172-5580-8 (v. 5: alk. paper)—
ISBN 0-7172-5581-6 (v. 6: alk. paper)—ISBN 0-7172-5582-4 (v. 7: alk. paper)—
ISBN 0-7172-5583-2 (v. 8: alk. paper)
        1. Health—Juvenile literature. 2. Health behavior—Juvenile literature. [1. Health.] I. Grolier Educational (Firm)

RA777 H386 2002
613—dc21
                                                                                2001040248

Contents

Volume 1: Addiction: Tobacco, Alcohol, and Other Drugs

v Introduction

7 Healthy Living: Teen Choices and Actions

12 Who Me? Check It Out!

19 Just the Facts: Addiction: Tobacco, Alcohol, and Other Drugs A to Z

Abstinence
Addiction
Addiction and Prescription
  Drugs
Addiction, Causes of
Addiction, Genetics and
Addiction, Injuries and
Addiction, Medications for
Addiction, Signs of
Addiction, Stages of
Advertising and Media
Al-Anon
Alateen
Alcohol
Alcohol Abuse
Alcohol Addiction
Alcohol Addiction, Causes of
Alcohol and Drug Counseling
Alcohol and Drug Rehabili-
  tation Programs
Alcohol and Drugs,
  Malnutrition and
Alcohol and Drugs, Mood
  and
Alcohol and Drugs, Sex and
Alcohol and Health Problems
Alcohol and Violence
Alcohol, Drug/Medication
  Interactions with
Alcohol Experimentation
Alcoholic Blackout
Alcoholics Anonymous (AA)
Alcoholism
Alcoholism Treatment
Alcohol Laws
Alcohol, Metabolism of
Alcohol Overdose
Alcohol Poisoning

Alternative Medicine
Amphetamines
Amyl Nitrate
Anabolic Steroids
Antabuse
Antibiotics
Antismoking Laws
Antismoking Products
Asthma
Barbiturates
Beer
Binge Drinking
Blood Alcohol Levels
Bronchitis
Cancers
Carcinogens
Centers for Disease Control
  and Prevention (CDC)
Child Abuse
Cirrhosis
Club Drugs
Cocaine
Codependency
Crack Cocaine
Date Rape Drugs
Death from Addictions
Delirium Tremens (DTs)
Dependence, Physical
Dependence, Psychological
Depressants
Designer Drugs
Detoxification
Domestic Violence and
  Abuse
Drinking in College
Driving while Intoxicated or
  Drug Impaired
Drug Abuse

Drug Addiction
Drug Enforcement Adminis-
  tration (DEA)
Drug-Free Zones
Drug Interactions
Drug Laws
Drug Overdose
Drugs
Drugs and Health Problems
Drug Testing
Ecstasy
Emphysema
Epidemiology
Fetal Alcohol Syndrome (FAS)
Freebasing
Hallucinations
Hallucinogens
Hashish
Heart Disease
Help–911
Hepatitis
Heroin
High Blood Pressure
HIV
Huffing
Hypnotherapy
Illegal Drugs
Inhalants
Injections
Intoxication
Intravenous Use of Illegal
  Drugs
LSD
Lung Cancer
Mainlining
Marijuana
Mescaline
Methadone

Methamphetamine
Naltrexone
Narcotics
Nicotine Replacement
  Therapy
Nonprescription Drugs
Nutrition and Drug Use
Opiates
Oral Cancer
PCP
Peer Pressure and Addiction
Pregnancy and Tobacco,
  Alcohol, and Drugs
Psychoactive Drugs
Psychosis
Raves
Secondhand Smoke
Smokeless Tobacco
Smoking Cessation
Stimulants
Support Groups
Surgeon General's Warnings
Teens and Addiction
Throat Cancer
Tobacco
Tobacco Addiction
Tobacco and Health
  Problems
Tobacco and Respiratory
  Diseases
Tobacco, Chemicals in
Tobacco, Forms of
Tobacco Laws
Tobacco Settlements
Tolerance, Physical
Twelve-Step Program
Withdrawal
Zero Tolerance Laws

153 Concerns and Fears

161 It Can't Happen to Me

166 Straight Talk

172 Directory of Services, Organizations, Help Sites, and Hotlines

174 Glossary

180 Further Reading and Internet Sites

183 Set Index

Introduction

What is the greatest threat to my health? If I begin smoking, will I be able to quit? Am I at risk of acquiring HIV infection and AIDS? How dangerous is it to ride in a car with a driver who has been drinking? Do I need to take vitamins to be healthy? How much sun does it take to cause skin cancer? Will crack cocaine hurt me if I just try it one time?

Such questions are typical of what people ask themselves regarding their health. We are constantly faced with making decisions that will affect our health and safety. This eight-volume reference set, *Health Matters!,* provides answers to myriad health-related questions by offering accurate and straightforward information on health topics ranging from addiction to environmental poisoning to infectious and chronic diseases. These volumes are also a valuable tool for conducting research, writing papers, and getting answers to personal questions about health and your body.

Over the past 30 years, in my capacity as a public school teacher and university professor, I have had the opportunity to work with teenagers, teachers, and librarians. As a head of national health and medical organizations I have also worked with surgeon generals, U.S. secretaries for health, and congressional leaders to help improve the health of all Americans.

As general editor of this encyclopedia I have drawn not only on these experiences but also on my experience as a member of the writing team that developed the *National Health Education Standards*—guidelines that define what students need to know and do to become health literate. Additionally, my contribution to these volumes reflects more than 30 years' participation in the development of the federal government's *Healthy People* initiatives outlined most recently in *Healthy People 2010,* a framework of national health objectives published by the U.S. Department of Health and Human Services.

Health Matters! blends the science and practice of disease prevention and health promotion with the daily concerns and decisions facing American teenagers and adults of all ages. I hope these volumes will answer your questions about health-related matters and arm you with the knowledge you need to make lifelong healthy decisions.

William M. Kane
General Editor

How to Use This Book

Health Matters! contains up-to-date information about the many topics and issues related to health and wellness—including addiction; mental health; sexuality and pregnancy; physical activity, weight and eating disorders; injuries and violence; environment poisoning; HIV infection, AIDS, and sexually transmitted diseases; and diseases and disabling conditions. The content in the set addresses all the issues and topics contained in the *National Health Education Standards* for achieving health literacy.

The set is divided into eight volumes, each focusing on a specific health-related topic. Within each volume the information is organized into six different sections. "Healthy Living: Teen Choices and Actions" prompts readers to consider the effect that their actions can have on their future health and life. "Who Me? Check It Out!" offers short quizzes that readers can use to assess how their current behaviors may affect their health. The heart of each volume, "Just the Facts," is an alphabetical encyclopedia of entries that provide in-depth facts and information young researchers need. "Concerns and Fears" looks at various issues that are of particular concern to teens. In "It Can't Happen to Me" readers will find stories about teenagers who have faced difficult health problems and struggled to overcome them. The final section, "Straight Talk," provides honest answers to some of the hard questions about health issues that students typically ask of adults.

Darrell Kozlowski and Charles Roebuck
Editors

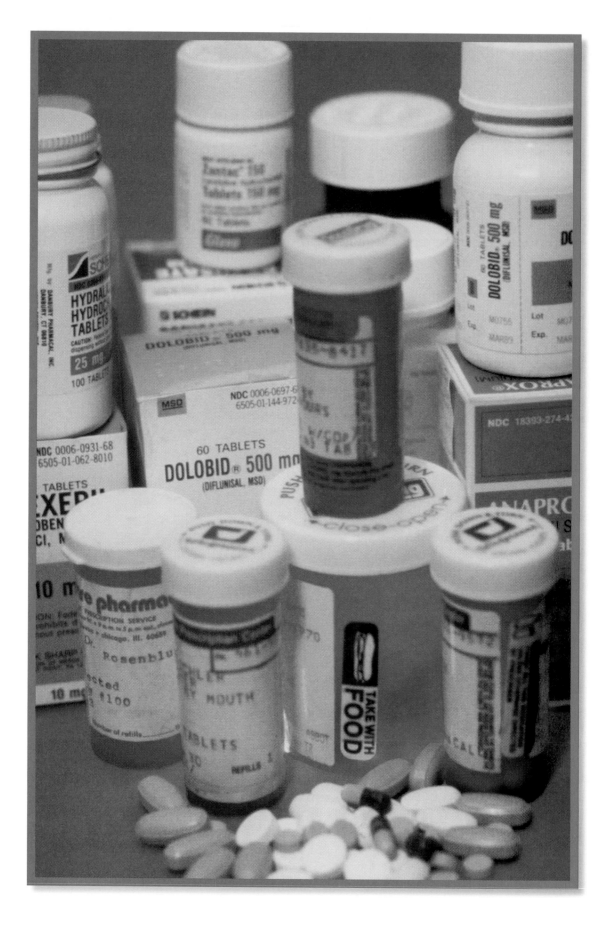

Healthy Living: Teen Choices and Actions

Remember when everyone used to ask you, "What do you want to be when you grow up?" Maybe they should have asked, "What do you want to be *if you decide* to grow up?" With almost every action you take today you choose not only who you will be today, tomorrow, and in five or ten years, but whether you will be at all.

First, the bad news: The best choices for you can be the hardest to make, and some of the teenagers you know today will die before they reach age 25 because they don't make positive choices.

For example, many teens die each year in car crashes involving the use of ALCOHOL, and teen drinking increases the chances of accidental injury or death. According to Substance Abuse and Mental Health Services Administration (SAMHSA), underage drinking led to approximately 11,322 nonfatal burns, 126 fatal burns, 1,420 near-drownings, and 208 drownings in just one year. Underage drinking was also a factor in approximately 1,200 homicides, 100,000 rapes, 83,000 robberies, 639,000 assaults, and 60,000 cases of child abuse. What's more, ALCOHOL ABUSE is linked to various health problems, some of which may be life-threatening.

The good news? You have the power to shape your life (to some extent) and ensure a happy and fulfilling life. In fact, you may have already made choices that will help ensure good emotional and physical health and affect the person you will be at age 25.

But I'm young, you say. And right now you feel pretty good most of the time, and you have plenty of energy. It may be hard to imagine any of this changing. Why think about it now? Look around. You may know kids who do not feel so good, or who take lots of risks. The top three killers of Americans ages 15–24 are accidents, suicide, and homicide.

That may make the choices for the next five or ten years seem pretty easy. Assuming you are basically healthy, all you have to do is avoid risky activities and not kill yourself. Right? But what about the less obvious choices, decisions that make you who you are—and who you will be in ten years—choices like who your friends are, how long you stay in school, what you do for fun?

Imagine describing yourself this way at 25: "I work for the airlines as a flight attendant. It's a great job because although I work long hours, I also have blocks of several days off at a time. During my free days I sleep late, date many different people, and party a lot. I like to drink and do a few drugs. My life is great!" Does this sound good? If it does, here is the part you failed to consider: Because of some choices you made along the way, you are close to becoming addicted to alcohol or DRUGS, are at increased risk of getting a sexually transmitted disease, are more likely to be injured or killed in an automobile crash as a result of drunk driving, and can barely pay your bills.

Consider this alternative: "I'm moving up in my job, but I still have plenty of free time. I hike on weekends, go to movies and dinner with friends, and work out three times a week at the gym. I don't do drugs and drink only occasionally at social gatherings. I'm not married yet, but that's my choice. I'm going out with a really great person now!" The part you failed to mention, because you are too modest, is that you're saving money, have bought a small condo, and have been putting money away for your retirement.

Okay, both scenarios are extremes. The point is, the choices you make *right now,* every day, are heading you in one direction or the other.

SAFE BEHAVIORS ARE SMART CHOICES

You can probably make some good guesses about which behaviors—ways you choose to act based on your own values—will keep you headed in the direction you want to go. (You also can choose your actions, which are the specific things you do that make up your patterns of behavior.) The tough part is making the smart choices about behavior, then acting on them.

According to the Joint Council on National Health Education Standards, which define what kids ought to know and be able to do, the first safe behavior is making smart choices when it comes to your body and mind, choices based on solid, reliable information. The other safe behaviors, in a nutshell, are exercising, eating right, reducing stress, and getting medical help when you need it.

Making the best choices for your own body and mind is mainly about being informed and thinking things through. Say that you're feeling very tired and unhappy lately. You haven't been sleeping or eating well, and you are having trouble concentrating in school and feel that your life is worthless. Your friends are concerned about you; one friend gives you a book about depression. You read that depression is a serious problem among teens—one that can be treated successfully. Your friends are very supportive and encourage you to seek professional help. You do, and soon your life and outlook begin to improve.

How about exercise? Here's a news flash: Dancing once a week for three hours, playing a game of pickup football or basketball a few times a week, or biking ten minutes to school is not

enough. The secret to feeling as good in ten years as you do right now is *vigorous activity that lasts at least 20 minutes at a time at least three times a week* (for instance, fast walking, jogging, biking, or swimming). *Plus* regular exercise *every day,* such as participation in physical education, games, or sports.

Exercise is just as important as eating right. Making smart choices about food might seem simple, but lots of people find it difficult. First, the simple part: Eat lots of fruits and vegetables; cut down on fried, fatty (red meat, cheese), and sugar-rich foods; and get informed about good nutrition (everything to do with how you eat and how your body uses food). Here are two examples of eating choices some would find hard: Grab a few donuts for breakfast every day, or sit down and have cereal and juice? You no doubt know what the *best* choice is, but how often will you make that choice? Given the choice of chocolate cake or a baked apple for dessert, how often will you choose the baked apple? (Check out "Healthy Eating Tips" at www.cdc.gov/nccdphp/dnpa/heal_eat.htm. The CENTERS FOR DISEASE CONTROL AND PREVENTION (CDC) web site is a great resource for all kinds of information on health and disease.)

Starting to feel stressed from thinking about all these choices? Fine. Stress is natural (it's a physical, chemical, or emotional factor that causes tension in the mind or body). Stress can come from positive *and* negative events in life—such as arguments, changing schools, moving, a big date, falling in love, the death of a pet or a person, feeling left out, or winning a prize. You can probably guess the best way to cope with stress—relax. The least stressed people spend time every week—or every day—doing whatever it is that they find relaxing—perhaps reading a book, taking a walk, meditating, or practicing yoga.

The last area of safe behavior calls for arranging a visit to the doctor, therapist, or another health professional when you suspect something is wrong with you. Say you have an oddly shaped mole that you're afraid is skin cancer. Perhaps you've been having weird thoughts or feelings and are worried that you're mentally ill. Or maybe you have genital itching, and you feel both embarrassed and worried that it might be from a sexually transmitted disease, or STD. (A sexually transmitted disease is an infection passed from person to person by intimate sexual contact.) If your condition is a serious one, the smart choice is to find out its cause—*now*. Medical tests can detect many diseases and problems early. Serious diseases like diabetes, heart disease, HIV, and many kinds of cancer can be fought more effectively if treatment starts early. Likewise, mental and emotional problems benefit from early diagnosis and treatment.

RISKY BEHAVIORS AND ACTIONS

You knew this section was coming, right? If there are safe behaviors and smart choices likely to keep you alive and well for the next decade, there are also unsafe ones. And there is a fact that intelligent people like to ignore: A person can be very smart and still make dumb choices, including choosing to practice risky behaviors.

The U.S. Centers for Disease Control and Prevention (CDC) (the main federal agency charged with protecting health and safety) lists **six risky behavior categories.**

Poor Diet. Here is what can lie ahead for people with consistently poor eating habits—people who are careless about what food they eat or who eat too much or too little. Eating certain foods—raw eggs, for instance (say, in uncooked cookie dough)—raises your chances of getting

sick from the bacteria or other toxic agents in those foods. There are more than 250 diseases that food carries. Food-borne illnesses include cholera, salmonella, typhoid fever, and gastroenteritis (severe diarrhea and vomiting). Related outcomes, besides death, include spontaneous abortion and blood poisoning.

Lack of Exercise. Obesity (usually weighing 20 percent or more of the expected weight for a given height) affects almost every area of life, from ordinary activity to sports, from self-confidence to energy levels to the kinds of clothes we can buy. Overweight people are at greater risk for stroke, heart disease, or osteoporosis. During a stroke an artery in the brain ruptures or gets clogged, causing paralysis (not being able to move) or death. Osteoporosis is a progressive loss of bone mass, which increases the risk of bone breakage, usually for older people. *But beginning in childhood,* people who get too little calcium put themselves at serious risk for the disease.

Eating disorders like anorexia and bulimia can be even more dangerous than simple overeating. Of 40 teenagers you know, one probably eats far too little (anorexia) or binges on food and then purges by vomiting or taking laxatives (bulimia). Anorexia can damage a person's heart, liver, and kidneys. The vomiting of bulimia often causes constant stomach pain, damage to the stomach and kidneys, and tooth decay. Both anorexia and bulimia can be fatal.

While people with bulimia often exercise too much, what about people who get too little

Six Risky Behavior Categories
POOR DIET
LACK OF EXERCISE
SMOKING
ACTIONS THAT LEAD TO UNINTENTIONAL AND INTENTIONAL INJURIES
ALCOHOL OR DRUG ABUSE
SEXUAL PRACTICES THAT INCREASE THE RISK OF STDS, HIV INFECTION, AND UNINTENDED PREGNANCY

exercise? They risk harm from all the conditions associated with poor diet and obesity, and also from high blood pressure, noninsulin-dependent diabetes, cancers, high cholesterol, back pain, feelings of stress, anxiety, and depression.

Smoking. For every teenager, smoking is almost guaranteed to have bad short-term health effects—damage to the respiratory system, addiction to nicotine, and some risk of other drug use. Statistics from the American Cancer Society and the CDC show that if you smoke regularly now, as a teenager, you will probably smoke throughout adulthood. *Then* you can count on *long-term* health consequences. Compared to nonsmokers, smokers are more likely to:

- Die seven years younger
- Die from lung cancer (if you are male, 22 times more likely; if you are female, 12 times more likely)
- Die from bronchitis and emphysema (males and females are at ten times the risk)
- Die from cardiovascular disease, such as heart attack or strokes, (both males and females are at three times the risk)

Unintentional and Intentional Injuries. Few people are injured or killed as a result of accidents, which are random events that cannot be prevented. Most are victims of unintentional injuries, which are almost always the direct result of actions that can be avoided, such as drinking and driving. Intentional injuries, which result from acts of violence, can also be prevented by identifying potentially dangerous situations ahead of time and taking action to avoid those risks.

Alcohol or Drug Abuse. There is no good news about drinking alcohol or using illegal drugs. And the earlier kids start drinking, the more likely they will be to develop a problem with alcohol or drugs later in life (look at www.kidshealth.org/teen for good information on all health issues). Teens who drink are more likely to be sexually active and to have unsafe, unprotected sex. When they drink, they may find it harder to resist unwanted sexual advances, and they are more vulnerable to sexual assault. Resulting pregnancies and STDs can change—or even end—lives.

The most widely used illegal drug in the United States is marijuana, which is often called a "gateway drug" because frequent smoking can lead to the use of stronger drugs. Marijuana is as tough on your lungs as cigarettes—steady smokers often suffer coughs, wheezing, and frequent colds. Of all abused substances, inhalants are the most likely to cause severe toxic reaction and death. Inhalants include glues, paint thinners, dry-cleaning fluids, gasoline, felt-tip marker fluid, correction fluid, hair spray, and spray paint. *Using inhalants, even one time, can kill you.*

Risky Sexual Practices. Equally harmful are HIV/AIDs and other infectious diseases. About one in four people between the ages of 15 and 55 will get an STD. Some can lead to long-term problems such as infertility (the inability to have a baby or father one) or even death if they are left untreated. STDs include chlamydia, genital herpes, genital warts, gonorrhea, hepatitis, HIV/AIDS, pubic lice (crabs), and syphilis.

Today, most adolescents infected with HIV are exposed to the virus through sexual intercourse or injection drug use, according to NIAID (National Institute of Allergy and Infectious Diseases). HIV, which causes AIDS, is the sixth leading cause of death for U.S. young people 15 to 24 years of age. *Most young adults with AIDS were likely infected with HIV as adolescents*, because the average period of time from HIV infection to the development of AIDS is ten years. Almost 18 percent of all reported cases of AIDS in the United States have occurred in people between the ages of 20 and 29.

WHAT'S TO COME
The rest of this book is packed with almost everything you ever wanted to know about addiction, tobacco, alcohol, and other drugs. In

the next section, "Who Me? Check It Out!" you will find tools to assess your own risk-taking behaviors. In "Just the Facts" are definitions of these topics, ranging from *abstinence* to *zyban*. That is followed by a section that addresses some of the typical "Concerns and Fears" that teenagers have about tobacco, alcohol, and other drugs. The section called "It Can't Happen to Me" includes stories of teenagers to whom some of these bad things and problems *did* happen. And in the final section, "Straight Talk," you will find honest answers to some of the hard questions about drugs and additions.

Special feature boxes provide health updates, help readers determine fact from folklore, focus on health-related behaviors in which teens are at special risk, and explore sensitive topics about which experts disagree or teens often lack understanding. The back of each volume contains a comprehensive glossary that gathers and defines keywords from all volumes; a list for further reading and Internet sites that suggests opportunities for additional research; and a

directory of health-related services, organizations, help sites, and hotlines. Finally, a set index will help the reader locate topics and terms through all eight volumes.

Health Matters! also provides a number of helpful reference features. Difficult words are printed in boldface type and defined in margin boxes as keywords. Cross-references that appear in small capital letters refer the reader to another entry in the same volume. Cross-references that appear in boldface and in small capital letters define the word as a keyword and also refer the reader to another entry in the same volume. Boldfaced and italicized cross-references, followed by a volume and number, lead the reader to related information that appears in another volume in the set. At the end of many entries "see also" cross-references point the reader to entries with related information in the same volume. Finally, some entries may also be followed by "More Sources," listing web sites that contain information related to the topic of the entry.

Who Me? Check It Out!

For many people the hard part about examining their risky behaviors is that once they have really looked at them, it is even harder to deny that they are choosing to behave in ways that put their mental health and happiness—and maybe even their life—in danger.

The choices are as simple as these: Which is more important, having a good time trying different drugs with my friends or avoiding bad habits that can seriously damage my health? Would I rather *be cool* by doing drugs to fit in or *be strong* by standing up for myself and how I want to live? Should I make someone angry by refusing to get in their car when they have been drinking, or should I risk getting killed in an ac-

cident? Is it better to *get wasted* so I can feel more comfortable at a party or to *keep my head* so I don't do something I'll regret?

All of the behaviors in the following reality checks are things *you* control. You can decide to do them or decide not to. No one can do the reality checks for you, and no one needs to know your answers. You are the only person who knows what you are really doing, thinking, and feeling. And naturally, you are also the person in charge of making positive changes if you decide you need to.

Read the following questions, and determine the answer that best describes your behavior. Keep track of your answers on a separate sheet of paper.

REALITY CHECK 1

What Are My Risks for Alcohol or Drug Abuse?

1. In the past 30 days did you get into a car with a driver who had been drinking alcohol?
   Yes   No

2. In the past 30 days did you operate any type of motor vehicle (car, bus, motorcycle, etc.) after you consumed alcohol?
   Yes   No

3. Have you had one or more drinks of alcohol in the past month?
   Yes   No

4. Have there been one or more times in the past 30 days when you drank five or more drinks of alcohol within a couple of hours?
   Yes   No

5. Have you ever used Ecstasy, LSD, mescaline or other hallucinogenic drugs?
   Yes   No

6. In the past 30 days have you sniffed or inhaled any household products, paints, or other forms of spray for the purpose of getting high?
   Yes   No

7. In the past 30 days have you used marijuana?
   Yes   No

8. Have you ever used a needle to inject an illegal drug into yourself?
   Yes   No

9. Have you ever used any anabolic steroids? (Sometimes used to build up muscles)
   Yes   No

Check Yourself

If you answered "yes" to . . .

Question 1 and 2: You are risking death or serious injury—to yourself and others. Even if you're alone in the car when you're drunk, you could hit an innocent pedestrian, bicyclist, or people in another car.

Question 3: If you have been drinking on several occasions, you risk developing an alcohol habit, which could develop into an addiction. You also risk being arrested if you are drinking alcohol and are under age 21.

Question 4: Drinking five or more drinks in a short period is called "binge drinking." You risk suffering from heart attack or even death. You also risk causing or being a victim of sexual assault.

Question 5: Hallucinogenic drugs put you at risk for heart attack, stroke, or mental illness. You have a much higher risk of injury or death.

Question 6: Inhalants can be extremely dangerous even the first time you try them. The risk is death or brain damage. Severe nosebleeds are also common.

Question 7: If you use marijuana even a few times a month, you could develop a physical or psychological need for the drug. You also risk respiratory diseases and cancer, as well as being jailed, since marijuana is an illegal drug.

Question 8: Injecting illegal drugs with shared needles can result in the transmission of diseases, including HIV. It is also a sign of addiction.

Question 9: Anabolic steroids are illegal unless a physician prescribes them for a growth deficiency. They can cause long-term physical and psychological problems.

Debriefing Reality Check 1

You know a little about the risks associated with the actions described in the questions. This section provides more details about those risks.

Questions 1 and 2: You risk your health and your life when you drink and drive or get inside a vehicle driven by a drunk driver.

Alcohol-impaired drivers can maim or kill themselves or others. Alcohol is involved in about a third of all motor vehicle crashes that result in injuries. Also, car crashes are the primary cause of death in the United States among people ages 15–24.

Even if no one is hurt, a drunk driver could be stopped by a police officer for speeding or for another infraction. This could result in losing a driver's license if the officer detects any signs of alcohol use.

Question 3: People under age 21 who drink alcohol risk becoming addicted to alcohol. Studies show that people who wait until they are 21 to drink alcohol have a much lower rate of alcoholism than those who start drinking when they are teenagers. It's also true that if you drink alcohol, you have a much higher risk of cross-addiction—that is abusing illegal drugs or becoming addicted to tobacco.

Question 4: If you answered "yes" to this question, you might be a binge drinker. For men binge drinking is defined as having five or more drinks in a row, and for women as having four or more drinks in a row. Binge drinkers are much more likely than others to get into fights, have unprotected sex, and get into trouble with the law. They also are in danger of "alcohol poisoning," in which the drinker consumers more than his or her body can tolerate. Alcohol poisoning can put you in the hospital and in some cases can result in death.

Question 5: If you answered "yes" to this question, you are heading for trouble unless you give up hallucinogenic drugs now. These drugs can cause heart attacks, mental illness, and brain damage, for starters.

Question 6: Inhalants have killed some people the first and only time they use them. Not everyone dies, though some people have long-term brain damage, headaches, and other severe side effects as a result of using inhalants. Even among chronic drug abusers it is usually younger teenage boys who use these substances the most.

Question 7: Many people think that marijuana is not dangerous. But this drug can be very potent today, and many people end up in emergency rooms after using the drug. Marijuana use in the teen years is predictive of continued drug abuse. Studies show that among those who first used marijuana at age 14 or younger, about 9 percent still used drugs as adults. Only 1.7 percent of adults who tried marijuana at age 18 or older continued to abuse the drug. Continued marijuana use can cause memory loss, panic attacks, and many health problems, including cancer.

Question 8: If you are injecting illegal drugs into yourself, then you are taking plenty of risks. The drug itself may kill you or make you severely ill. The needle that you shared with someone else could give you hepatitis or a sexually transmitted disease like HIV, which leads to AIDS. When you inject illegal drugs, you are an addict or in danger of becoming one.

Question 9: In the short term steroids may help build up muscle faster. But the risks are very great. Men who abuse steroids risk shrinking of their testicles and impotence. Women (and yes, there are some women who abuse steroids) risk disturbed menstrual periods and shrinking breasts. Both men and women risk experiencing infertility and severe psychotic rages.

Read the following questions, and determine the answer that best describes your behavior. Keep track of your answers on a separate sheet of paper.

REALITY CHECK 2

Do I Have a Tobacco-Addiction Problem?

1. Do you smoke cigarettes daily?
   Yes   No

2. Do you use any form of smokeless tobacco, including chewing tobacco or snuff or any product that contains tobacco but was not smoked?
   Yes   No

3. Do you smoke cigars and cigarillos (or little cigars) daily more than several times a week?
   Yes   No

4. Do most of your friends either smoke or use smokeless tobacco?
   Yes   No

5. Does smoking make you feel older or more mature?
   Yes   No

6. Do any members of your family smoke?
   Yes   No

Check Yourself

If you answered "yes" to . . .

Question 1: You are or soon will be addicted to cigarettes. You are risking bronchitis, cancer, emphysema, and other diseases.

Question 2: You may think smokeless tobacco is safer than cigarettes. You are wrong. Smokeless tobacco causes mouth and throat cancer as well as respiratory ailments.

Question 3: Cigars and cigarillos (little cigars) are also addictive and can cause cancer.

Question 4: If most or all of your friends smoke, then you may experience peer pressure to smoke too. Resisting the temptation to smoke is difficult, but it can be done.

Question 5: The only people who think that smoking makes them seem older or more mature are teenage smokers. If you keep smoking, it will make you look older because smoking can cause wrinkles to appear sooner than they would otherwise.

Question 6: If your family members smoke, you have a greater risk of smoking too. You also may be affected by secondhand smoke.

Debriefing Reality Check 2

This self-check is not about whether a behavior is right or wrong, or good or bad. It is about whether choosing a behavior is choosing to take a *risk*.

Question 1: If you are smoking every day, there isn't any question about it—you are addicted to tobacco. Although it can be difficult, you can quit smoking. Check with your doctor for safe ways to rid yourself of the need for tobacco.

Tobacco is the primary preventable cause of death in the United States. It causes lung cancer, oral cancer, heart disease, and stroke. According to the Centers for Disease Control and Prevention, if current smoking patterns continue unchanged, 5 million people who were age 17 and under in 1995 will die prematurely as a result of smoking.

Question 2: Smokeless tobacco is highly addictive and is a cause of oral cancer. It is a contributing factor to cardiovascular disease. It also causes diseases of the teeth and gums. Many people are also repelled by the spitting that is prompted by smokeless tobacco.

Question 3: Cigars and cigarillos are not safer than cigarettes. They cause cancer and bronchitis, and they cause your hair, skin, and clothes to smell of tobacco.

Question 4: It's hard to resist friends when they encourage you to smoke. You may think that since they do it, it's all right to smoke. The reality is that your friends are probably addicted. They don't like to think about that fact, however. Somehow, it may make it seem like an okay activity if their nonsmoking friends start to smoke too. But friends or other peers are harming you if they urge you to smoke, and you are endangering yourself if you give in to this peer pressure.

Question 5: The only people who think smoking makes them look older are teenagers who smoke. However, if you keep smoking, you will look older than you are, and by then you won't like it. Smoking tends to accentuate the fine lines on a person's face, around the eyes and around the cheeks. Smoking is also very bad for the skin, which is harmed by the constant accumulation of smoke.

Question 6: If people in your family think smoking is a normal thing to do, then it can be very difficult to *not* smoke. Moreover, you are already exposed to secondhand smoke, so why not go ahead and smoke? Bad choice.

You can tell other family members about the risks of cancer, emphysema, and bronchitis that they face, and you can name relatives and other people that they know who have sickened and died as a result of smoking or using smokeless tobacco. But the fact is, the only one you can really control is yourself.

Many people who are still smoking in their thirties and forties (and older) say that they started when they were 13 or 14—or younger. The addiction seems to take hold more strongly among users who start young. However, you are not doomed to smoke. It isn't easy to quit smoking, but it is certainly doable. Tell your parent or guardian that you would like to consult your physician about kicking the habit, whether through medication, hypnotherapy, or another method.

Just the Facts: Addiction: Tobacco, Alcohol, and Other Drugs A-Z

The first step in dealing effectively with a health problem is to understand it—to know enough about it to take appropriate action and to prevent it from happening again if possible. Reliable health information can also give you a sense of control over the situation and ease unwarranted fears. Without this information you are at the mercy of biological processes. You can only wait to see what happens.

This section provides you with knowledge that will help you take charge and live a safer life. Its entries contain reliable information about tobacco, alcohol, and other drugs. You'll learn about the use of tobacco and alcohol and the various problems and health risks associated with these substances. You'll also learn about other legal and illegal drugs, the various medici-nal or recreational purposes of them, and the potential dangers of drug use and abuse. In addition to learning how drugs affect users physically and psychologically after both short-term and long-term use, you'll also learn about the risks of becoming addicted to drugs.

Perhaps most importantly, the information in this section will help you decrease the risks associated with the abuse of alcohol, tobacco, and other drugs. You'll learn how to avoid danger-ous situations and how to make better decisions when confronted with opportunities to try these substances. In short, this section contains some-thing that is often difficult for teens to find—up-to-date and useful facts based on the best scien-tific and medical information available.

ABSTINENCE Complete avoidance of a substance or behavior. In terms of ALCOHOL or DRUGS abstinence refers to the avoidance of alcohol, ILLEGAL DRUGS, or legal drugs such as TOBACCO. Absti-nence from alcohol is a central part of the program of ALCOHOLICS ANONYMOUS (AA). Some people, however, argue that such absti-nence is not necessary and that moderation in drinking is possible. Most experts disagree with this argument, as do members of AA and AL-ANON. AA believes that, for an alcoholic, any amount of alcohol will always lead to out-of-control drinking. [*See also* TWELVE-STEP PROGRAM.]

ACID See LSD.

ADDICTION The physical and psychological need for substances such as ALCOHOL, DRUGS, and TOBACCO. According to the National Institute on Drug Abuse, addiction is a *chronic disease* (see Volume 8)—that is, it lasts a long time and is difficult to cure. Characteristics of addiction include compulsive drug seeking and use; chemical changes in the brain; and **relapse**, a return to using an addicting substance after an attempt to give it up.

Addiction affects millions of people in the United States and around the world. In 1999 some 8 million Americans were addicted to alcohol and over 3 million to ILLEGAL DRUGS. Of these about 1.5 million required both drugs and alcohol. Additionally, 57 million Americans were addicted to cigarettes, with millions more hooked on other tobacco products, such as cigars, SMOKELESS TOBACCO, and pipe tobacco.

Symptoms of Addiction. Like all diseases, addiction has certain symptoms. All addicts display most of these symptoms, particularly the major ones.

Craving. Addicts are possessed by an intense desire, or craving, for addictive substances. It is a craving that addicted people cannot ignore. Thus addicts cannot stop drinking, taking drugs, or smoking, nor can they limit the amounts that they consume. They lose all control; this loss of control is known as **substance abuse**.

Addicts sometimes find their substance abuse temporarily stopped by forces that are no more under their control than their craving for alcohol, drugs, or tobacco. For example, a determined friend or family member or a lack of money may block an addict from getting the addictive substance. Abuse can also end for a time when an addict becomes sick or passes out. Still, the craving, along with lack of control, remains.

Tolerance. Another symptom of addiction is physical **tolerance**, which creates a need for greater amounts of alcohol, drugs, or tobacco. This increased need for the substance is necessary in order to attain the same high as in the past. Thus an alcoholic moves from a few drinks to a whole bottle, and an addicted smoker from half a pack of cigarettes to two or three packs a day.

Preoccupation. Addicts are preoccupied with getting their addictive substances. They will spend large chunks of time and money in this quest. They will even lie, cheat, steal, or commit other crimes to get the substance they crave.

Physical Dependence. A final major symptom of addiction is physical dependence. Addicts deprived of tobacco, alcohol, or

relapse a return to using an addictive substance after attempting to give it up
substance abuse excessive use of alcohol, drugs, tobacco, or other addictive substances
tolerance capacity of the body to endure or become less responsive to a substance with repeated use

drugs will exhibit a wide range of physical responses. They may sweat, develop headaches, or have seizures. At worst, they may lapse into a coma or die.

Withdrawal. All of these physical reactions are caused by WITH-DRAWAL from the addictive substance. Whether addicts are drinkers, drug users, or smokers, those who want to kick their habits have to face withdrawal and the symptoms associated with it.

Never easy, withdrawal is more dangerous to some addicts than others. Where the smoker may be irritable and anxious, the alcoholic may face the life-threatening DELIRIUM TREMENS (DTs), with its seizures and HALLUCINATIONS. The drug addict may also experience seizures, hallucinations, and PSYCHOSIS during withdrawal.

Addiction and the Family. Addicts do not bear the cost of their addiction alone. Their families often pay a heavy price as well. Experts note that most cases of CHILD ABUSE and *domestic violence and abuse* (see Volume 5) are directly related to alcohol or drug use. In many cases the abuser is addicted to these substances.

Addiction and Crime. Addiction has other social consequences besides child and domestic abuse. Many addicts find that they cannot earn enough money to pay for their habits, so they turn to crime. Their crimes range from petty theft all the way to murder. Many adolescent addicts also become criminals. For example, among adolescents ages 12–17, MARIJUANA users are twice as likely as nonusers to steal, attack others, and destroy property. [*See also* DEPENDENCE, PHYSICAL; TOLERANCE, PHYSICAL.]

ADDICTION AND MENTAL HEALTH See Volume 2.

ADDICTION AND PEER PRESSURE See PEER PRESSURE AND ADDICTION.

ADDICTION AND PRESCRIPTION DRUGS Legal drugs that can lead to ADDICTION, which should be obtained from a druggist and with a doctor's permission. However, people who abuse or become addicted to prescription drugs get them both legally and illegally.

Legal Abuse and Addiction. Most people who take prescription medications take them responsibly. However, many prescribed medications, particularly sedatives or painkillers, are addictive if used improperly. With such medications people build up a tolerance to the drugs that leads to addiction. Medications that are potentially very addictive are BARBITURATES, often prescribed to help people sleep, and narcotic painkillers such as Vi-

The Price of Addiction
According to *Healthy People 2010,* a report by the U.S. Department of Health and Human Services, addiction comes with a heavy price tag. An estimated 430,000 people die each year from related illnesses due to TOBACCO ADDICTION alone. Another 100,000 die from diseases and conditions related to ALCOHOL ABUSE and addiction. Finally, some 12,000 abusers of ILLEGAL DRUGS die each year from AIDS contracted from dirty needles, or syringes. In sum, addictions kill more than a half million people in the United States each year.

What about OxyContin?

When it became available to the public in 1995, the powerful new synthetic drug OxyContin was hailed by health care professionals as a major breakthrough in the treatment of debilitating and chronic pain. For many patients who could not find pain relief from other medications, OxyContin seemed to be a godsend. Sales of the drug skyrocketed, and it soon became one of the most popular drugs on the market. Within two years, however, stories became to circulate about the illegal use and abuse of OxyContin, as well as a number of deaths associated with the drug. News of an OxyContin "epidemic" also brought attention to the potential for the abuse of prescription drugs. However, much of this news was not based on accurate or reliable information. While levels of OxyContin abuse were rising, the actual dangers were overblown—especially when measured against the benefits of the drug in the fight against pain. Unfortunately for many chronic pain sufferers, the controversy surrounding OxyContin has dramatically curtailed its use, even though the drug remains one of the most effective pain medications yet discovered.

codin. Abuse of prescription drugs may occur accidentally when a patient doesn't follow the instructions provided by his or her doctor or druggist.

Illegal Abuse and Addiction. Some prescription drug abusers acquire their drugs by getting a legal prescription drug for non-medical use. People receive these drugs in a number of ways, including *doctor shopping*, in which the person keeps changing doctors so they can obtain enough of the drug to feed their addiction. By frequently changing doctors, the user makes it harder for doctors to recognize that they have already been prescribed the drug and are abusing it. Another way people obtain prescription drugs illegally is by buying the drug from a legitimate patient in need of the medication. For example, one disturbing trend occuring in many schools is that students with ***attention deficit hyperactivity disorder (adhd)*** (see Volume 2) are selling their prescription Ritalin drugs to make a profit from classmates.

Epidemiology. The National Institute of Drug Abuse (NIDA) says that prescription drug abuse in the United States occurs most often among older adults, adolescents, and women. According to their 2001 report on prescription drugs, 17 percent of adults ages 60 and older may be abusing prescription medications. Older persons use more prescription drugs than most people, placing them at a greater risk for dependence and addition.

The Effects of Prescription Drug Abuse. Prescription drug abuse can have very harmful effects, depending on the type of drug. Opioids, which include pain killers such as morphine, codeine, OxyContin, and Demerol, may lead to severe respiratory problems and even death. Opioids are extremely addictive. As users develop a tolerance to the drug, they must take higher doses to get the same results.

CNS DEPRESSANTS, often used for anxiety and sleep disorders, include barbiturates and benzodiazepines such as Valium and Xanax. These drugs slow down brain activity so that when user stops taking them, their brain activity races out of control, which can cause seizures. Users can also develop a tolerance to CNS depressants after long-term use.

Stimulants such as Dexadrine and Ritalin encompass the third category of prescription drugs commonly abused. These drugs increase brain activity and are frequently used to treat ADHD and *depression* (see Volume 2). They are also prescribed for *narcolepsy*, a condition in which a person frequently falls asleep for brief periods of time. Stimulants increase blood pressure and heart rate, and, when abused, may cause cardiovascular failure or seizure.

Prevention. Healthcare providers should prescribe needed medications appropriately and try to identify prescription drug abuse when it exists. Screening for any type of substance abuse can be incorporated into routine history-taking with questions about what prescriptions and over-the-counter (OTC) medicines the patient is taking and why. Providers should look out for increases in the amount of a drug needed or frequent requests for refills. This may indicate that the patient has developed a degree of tolerance that could lead to addiction. After discovering abuse or addiction, a provider can help the patient recognize the problem, set goals for recovery, and seek treatment when necessary

Pharmacists should provide patients with clear information about how to take a medication appropriately, the effects the medication may have, and any possible DRUG INTERACTIONS. They can help prevent prescription fraud by looking for false or altered prescription forms. Many pharmacies have developed hotlines to alert other pharmacies in the area when fraud is detected. [See also TOLERANCE, PHYSICAL; TOLERANCE, PSYCHOLOGICAL.]

MORE SOURCES See www.nida.gov/drugpages/prescription; www.health.org/nongovpubs/prescription

ADDICTION AND TEENS See TEENS AND ADDICTION.

ADDICTION, CAUSES OF The numerous factors that give rise to ADDICTION. Nobody plans to become an addict, and nearly all who use addictive substances for the first time think that they will be able to control the use of them. Sadly, these people are often mistaken because experimentation can lead to continued use and then addiction.

People may be introduced to addictive substances by their friends or by family members. Older brothers and sisters have a major influence on their younger siblings; and if a big sister or brother uses DRUGS, ALCOHOL, or TOBACCO, so likely will the younger sibling.

Some substances are more rapidly addictive than others. CRACK COCAINE, for example, is almost instantly addictive. But even before addiction use of a substance may become continual because of the pleasurable feelings associated with it. Nicotine, for example, triggers a pleasurable response in the brain and body and makes users desire tobacco even before they are actually addicted. If use continues, this psychological attraction may then be followed by a physical need for the substance. At that point the person has become addicted.

ADDICTION, GENETICS AND Possible genetic factors that contribute to ADDICTION. Scientists are currently studying the ge-

netic code of humans. In part, they hope to discover how diseases, or predispositions to diseases, are inherited. Addictions to ALCOHOL, TOBACCO, and DRUGS may have such a genetic cause.

Several important research projects, such as the Collaborative Study on the Genetics of Alcoholism, have found evidence that **genes** for ALCOHOLISM are located on certain **chromosomes**—chromosomes 1 and 7 and possibly chromosome 2. Study of Native Americans in the Southwest has found evidence of a link between alcoholism and a gene on chromosome 11, as well as indications of a gene on chromosome 4 that may protect against alcoholism.

A genetic base for alcoholism has found further support in studies of twins raised apart and adopted children separated from their biological parents at a young age. There may also be genetic predispositions to ALCOHOL ABUSE and TOBACCO ADDICTION. Genes may also play a role in determining general addictive or impulsive behavior that leads to the abuse of alcohol, drugs, and tobacco.

Scientists, however, are fairly certain that no one gene causes a person to become an addict. It is more likely that several genes are involved. Moreover, the influence of the environment on addiction must be taken into account as well. For example, if a person with a genetic predisposition for addictive behavior is raised in a strict religious environment where drugs or alcohol are prohibited, would that person become an addict if he or she remains in that environment? If the person leaves the environment and begins using alcohol or drugs, would that trigger the underlying genetic predisposition to addictive behavior?

At this time it is difficult, if not impossible, to predict genetic predispositions to addictions. If people are drug or alcohol addicts, then their children may or may not become addicts. The question experts continue to ask themselves is: When the children of addicts become addicts themselves, is it because of genetics or because of environment? Or both? At this point no one knows for sure.

In the future, when genetics are better understood, it may be possible to change the genetic makeup of people as a way of treating illnesses and addictions. However, this topic is highly controversial for many reasons. For example, will genes be donated from other people, and if so, from whom? Will genes that are modified create other problems that experts can not yet foresee? These and other issues about *genetic engineering* (see Volume 8) are a major concern of scientists and others.

ADDICTION, INJURIES AND Accidental harm that results from using addictive substances. Individuals addicted to DRUGS or

Keywords

chromosomes threadlike bodies in the nuclei of living cells that carry genes
genes the part of living cells that carries specific characteristics and passes them on from one generation to the next
nicotine a toxic and highly addictive drug found in tobacco

ALCOHOL are more likely to be injured in car crashes or falls than nonaddicts. Likewise, alcoholics or drug abusers who use TOBACCO are more likely to be harmed by accidental fires than others. People who accompany an alcoholic or drug abuser also face an increased risk of *unintentional injuries* (see Volume 5) as a result of mishaps.

The chief reason for this increased risk is that alcohol and drugs impair the judgment and coordination and interfere with the senses of addicts. As a result, abusers are more likely to make serious errors that lead to injuries to themselves and to others. The use of alcohol also increases the probability that injuries will be more serious than if the person were sober. [*See also* DRIVING WHILE INTOXICATED OR DRUG IMPAIRED.]

ADDICTION, MEDICATIONS FOR Legally prescribed drugs that are used to help addicted individuals break their ADDICTION to ALCOHOL, DRUGS, or TOBACCO. In addition to aid provided through counseling and membership in self-help groups such as ALCOHOLICS ANONYMOUS (AA), addicted individuals may also find relief with certain medications.

Medications for Tobacco Addiction. Physicians prescribe a variety of drugs to help people overcome their addiction to tobacco. NICOTINE REPLACEMENT THERAPY, which actually provides a quantity of **nicotine**, is one solution that has worked to free many smokers of their habit. The nicotine comes in several forms: as gum, a skin patch, an inhaler, or a nasal spray.

Other drugs may help smokers give up tobacco as well. Zyban (bupropion) is a prescribed drug that has been proven effective in alleviating the desire to smoke. While doctors have also had success with other medications, so far Zyban is the only nonnicotine drug that the Food and Drug Administration has specifically approved for SMOKING CESSATION.

Medications for Alcohol Abuse. In the past ANTABUSE was the drug most used for its effect in creating an aversion to alcohol. The drug makes alcoholics violently ill even if they drink only a small amount of alcohol.

More recently, researchers and physicians have successfully treated ALCOHOL ADDICTION with NALTREXONE, a drug that acts on the brain to block the pleasure centers stimulated by alcohol. This means that alcoholics who take naltrexone and then drink will not feel the intense pleasure that they normally get from drinking alcohol.

Medications for Drug Abuse. Since about 1970 METHADONE has been the most common medication used to treat individuals addicted to HEROIN. Both methadone and heroin are NARCOTICS with similar effects on the body, including the potential for addiction. However, because methadone does not produce a euphoric high like heroin, it is considered the lesser evil. Additionally, some researchers have also reported success in treating heroin addicts, as well as those addicted to COCAINE, with a combination of Antabuse and another medication called buprenorphine.

ADDICTION, SIGNS OF Indicators that a person is addicted to ALCOHOL, DRUGS, or TOBACCO. There are usually a number of clear indicators of ADDICTION. One sign of addiction is that the person centers his or her life around making sure that the addictive substance is always readily available. To addicts the only two important issues are using the substance and getting more of it.

Relapse and Withdrawal. Another sign of addiction is *relapse*, a return to using an addictive substance after a failed attempt to give it up. A further sign is WITHDRAWAL, a series of physical symptoms suffered by addicts when they are off alcohol, drugs, or tobacco. For example, withdrawal from tobacco may cause headache, stomach pain, poor concentration, and irritability.

Physical Signs. Addiction also has physical signs that an outsider can readily see. These physical indicators vary considerably depending on the abused substance. For example, AMPHETAMINES tend to make people jumpy and irritable and cause them to overreact greatly to stimuli. DEPRESSANTS, on the other hand, are more likely to cause a person to be dull and sleepy. Dilated (enlarged) pupils of the eyes are a sign of addiction to COCAINE or HEROIN.

Behavioral Indicators. Addicts also exhibit behavioral changes. Often they lose most, if not all, interest in former activities. They may sleep much less or much more than in the past. They may eat far more or less than before. They may be constantly late to school or work, when that was not a pattern in the past. They may be quick to anger, more ready to argue, or have a more aggressive attitude.

Most frightening of all, addicts can become violent. For example, people addicted to ANABOLIC STEROIDS or AMPHETAMINES are given to rage and extreme suspicion of others.

ADDICTION, STAGES OF Progressive patterns of behavior that many addicts go through that lead to ADDICTION. An addiction may take a brief period to develop, or it could take years. Addiction to tobacco or COCAINE, for example, can be very rapid. Addiction to ALCOHOL can also develop quickly, but more commonly it takes years of heavy use to develop an ALCOHOL

ADDICTION. For other drugs the time from first use to the point of addiction varies.

When addiction is not immediate, there are usually identifiable stages that lead to the development of addiction. These include psychological dependence, tolerance, and physical dependence.

Psychological dependence occurs when a person has a desire or need for DRUGS, alcohol or TOBACCO. Without the substance the person may feel out of sorts and irritable. He or she may actively try to locate a supply of the substance. But the person will not suffer any physical reactions if he or she does not take the substance.

In the next stage of addiction a person develops a tolerance to a substance. This means that he or she requires more of the drug or alcohol than in the past. Instead of one drink being enough to change a person's mood, two or more drinks will be needed to provide the same effect.

Physical dependence is the final stage of addiction. By this point the body craves and needs the addictive substance. Without it the addicted person will suffer from physical symptoms of WITHDRAWAL, which may be mild or very severe. Some symptoms of withdrawal are heavy perspiration, vomiting, and stomach or headache. Severe withdrawal symptoms include HALLUCINATIONS and convulsions, which can lead to coma and death. [*See also* DEPENDENCE, PHYSICAL; DEPENDENCE, PSYCHOLOGICAL; TOLERANCE, PHYSICAL.]

ADVERTISING AND MEDIA Promotion of products in the popular media, including on television and radio, in magazines and newspapers, and in movies. For years ALCOHOL and TOBACCO have been advertised in various media.

It is illegal for people under age 18 to buy tobacco products, and they cannot consume alcohol legally until they are age 21. Nonetheless, many underage people do smoke and drink. One factor that may contribute to the use of these products by underage individuals is the influence of advertising and media, particularly corporate promotional attempts to portray drinking and smoking as fun-filled and glamorous activities practiced by good-looking young adults.

Advertising and media also affect how people regard ILLEGAL DRUGS. Because they are illegal for everyone to consume, regardless of age, these substances are not advertised. Yet the media are still involved to an extent in shaping the attitudes of young consumers to these as well as other addictive substances. Hollywood, television, and other media outlets can and do depict attractive movie stars smoking, abusing alcohol, and using both legal and illegal drugs in movies and on television.

In a study of the most popular videos rented in 1996 and 1997 researchers found that characters used alcohol in 93 percent of the movies and used tobacco in 89 percent. Illegal drugs such as MARI-JUANA or COCAINE were depicted in 22 percent of the movies. Further, an analysis of the 1,000 most popular songs in 1996 and 1997 found that 27 percent of the songs referred to using illegal drugs or alcohol. The underlying message received by many adolescents from advertising and the media is that these substances are normal and also, if you consume them, you will be more like the celebrities who use them.

Big Tobacco. The tobacco industry has been very successful in using the media to advertise and promote their products. They also spend heavily: In 1999 tobacco companies spent over $8 billion on advertising and promotion in the United States. They also relied heavily on billboards to promote their products until 1998, when the federal government banned tobacco companies from promoting cigarettes in billboard ads.

Targeting Youth. In the year 2000 the CENTERS FOR DISEASE CONTROL AND PREVENTION (CDC) estimated that the average 14-year-old had already been exposed to $20 billion in advertising and promotion specifically designed to create a positive image of tobacco products.

Some ads have targeted children and adolescents by using cartoon characters. The most famous of these was Joe Camel, a character that appealed to young people. Since Joe Camel was introduced in 1988, Camel's share of the adolescent cigarette market grew from under 1 percent to about 13 percent by 1993. In 1998, as part of a major lawsuit settlement between cigarette companies and the states that sued them, the R.J. Reynolds Company agreed to stop using Joe Camel and other cartoon characters to promote their products.

Targeting Women. Advertisers have been very successful at reaching specific groups who they hope will smoke. One very successful ad campaign, launched in the 1960s and directed at attracting women to smoke, used the slogan "You've Come a Long Way, Baby!" In the mid-1990s, "It's a woman thing" was another profitable promotion slogan in the campaign to sell cigarettes to females.

The underlying message of these advertising campaigns was that women who smoke are independent and empowered. Women are also depicted as slender and attractive. Tobacco companies advertise heavily in women's magazines; and research has indicated that when these magazines accept cigarette ads, they are less likely to publish antismoking articles.

Targeting Minority Groups. The tobacco industry has also targeted minority groups as smokers. Before agreeing to remove all tobacco billboards as part of a settlement with the federal government in 1998, the tobacco industry had placed numerous billboards in minority communities. One 1993 study, for example, found that the greatest number of tobacco billboards in San Diego were found in Asian American neighborhoods. The least number were found in white communities. The tobacco industry has also advertised very heavily in magazines oriented to African Americans. Most recently, the tobacco industry has targeted Native Americans, who are known heavy users of tobacco. Among the products promoted are American Spirit cigarettes, which are advertised as "natural." The product's package features an American Indian smoking a pipe.

Counteradvertising. Many states and private groups have used antismoking ads in recent years in an attempt to counteract years of prosmoking advertising and promotion. It appears to be having

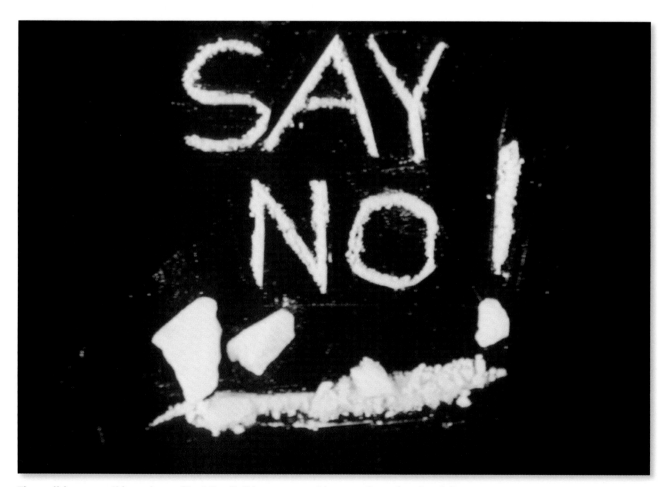

The well-known antidrug slogan "Just Say No" has appeared in many forms in advertising.

some effect, although these efforts are still relatively new. Most states have also committed money from TOBACCO SETTLEMENTS to spend on tobacco prevention.

Alcohol Advertising. At least a billion dollars is spent each year to advertise alcohol products. Although alcohol ads do not appear to target youth, they nonetheless have an effect on them. Many studies have shown that children and adolescents take note of alcohol ads and can correctly identify product brands by their ads. Studies have also shown that drinking habits are affected by advertisements. According to the research, children who are aware of these ads are more likely to consume alcohol as adults.

As with the tobacco companies, the alcohol industry also seeks to depict the consumption of alcohol as a fun activity undertaken by people who are beautiful, smart, and sophisticated. Beer appeals primarily to males; thus many beer ads feature an athletic-looking man engaging in active sports, often with a lovely, admiring woman nearby.

Most companies, of course, try to place their products in an extremely positive light and often depict their consumers as attractive and appealing people. The difference between most other products and tobacco and alcohol is that the latter are addicting for many people, and they also cost lives.

AL-ANON A SUPPORT GROUP for adults who have family members or friends who are alcoholics. Another important self-help group is ALATEEN, which is a branch of Al-Anon. Although not a part of ALCOHOLICS ANONYMOUS (AA), Al-Anon follows the TWELVE-STEP PROGRAM created by AA.

Most members of Al-Anon (96 percent) are 34 years old or over, and the majority (85 percent) are women. More than 77 percent of those who attend Al-Anon meetings are there because of a recommendation, often from a respected professional such as a therapist, doctor, or clergyperson.

Al-Anon provides an important psychological and emotional outlet for the family members and friends of alcoholics, many of whom blame themselves for the ALCOHOL ADDICTION. Some alcoholics tell family members or friends that they are at fault. The family members or friends may believe that if they were more attractive, better-behaved, richer, or had other qualities, the alcoholic would stop drinking. They may also believe that they should lie and cover up when the alcoholic does not show up for work or gets into trouble. This type of relationship or unspoken agreement between addicts and nonaddicts, which allows an addiction to continue unchallenged, is called CODEPENDENCY.

Participation in Al-Anon helps free family members of self-blame and guilt and teaches them that it is the alcoholic who must take responsibility for his or her drinking. The organization also gives people who may have suffered in silence for years with an alcoholic an opportunity to meet others who have had similar experiences. Realizing that they are not alone in their problem can be an enormous relief for most people. [*See also* ALCOHOL AND DRUG REHABILITATION PROGRAMS; ALCOHOLISM.]

ALATEEN A self-help organization for children and adolescents who have friends or relatives who are alcoholics. Alateen is a branch of AL-ANON, an organization for adults who have family members or friends who are suffering from ALCOHOLISM.

Most Alateen members are between ages 10 and 18, and the average age is 14. About two-thirds of members are female. Most of the young people who attend Alateen (about 90 percent) have a parent or stepparent who is an alcoholic. The majority of members (92 percent) become involved with Alateen because of personal recommendations from a professional, such as a doctor, therapist, or member of the clergy.

Alateen teaches members about alcoholism and offers understanding and compassion from others who have experienced the same problem. The organization is not connected to ALCOHOLICS ANONYMOUS (AA), but members also follow the TWELVE-STEP PROGRAM that is a major component of AA. [*See also* ALCOHOL AND DRUG REHABILITATION PROGRAMS.]

ALCOHOL A liquid made from distilled grains, fruits, or vegetables. Beer and wine are both forms of alcohol, as are rum, whiskey, and scotch and other distilled spirits. Wine coolers and mixed drinks are also forms of alcoholic beverages.

The alcoholic content of a beverage varies a great deal. Wine may contain about 12 percent alcohol, while beer may have 7 percent or less. Distilled forms of alcohol are measured by their proof—a number that is double the actual percentage of alcohol. For example, a bourbon whiskey that is 80 proof contains 40 percent alcohol.

Effects of Alcohol. Many people mistakenly believe that alcohol is a STIMULANT because it makes them feel happy. However, alcohol is actually a DEPRESSANT. It has a sedating, or slowing-down, effect on a person, and it lowers inhibitions, sometimes causing a person to behave in ways they would never normally act when sober.

Alcohol affects people differently, depending on such factors as their weight or the amount of food in their stomachs. Because thin people weigh less and have less blood, body tissue, and fluids than average-sized or heavier individuals, smaller amounts of alcohol will lead to INTOXICATION faster. If a person consumes a meal, the alcohol affects them more slowly than if they drink on an empty stomach. Other factors that affect the response to alcohol are the person's overall psychological state—happy/sad, elated/angry, and so forth—as well as whether they are tired from lack of sleep or feeling under stress.

Alcohol also has unpredictable effects on people. Some people, for example, become very angry or very sad when they are intoxicated. Others may become abusive to friends and family members. Still others become silly or sleepy if they drink.

Short-term Health Effects. Alcohol consumption can have short-term and long-term impacts. Some of the short-term effects of alcohol use are impaired senses and coordination and distorted judgment. People who drink may also have bad breath and experience vomiting and a hangover, with symptoms that may include headache and nausea. Because alcohol consumption impairs coordination and also delays response time, it is extremely dangerous to drink and drive.

Long-term Health Effects. People who abuse alcohol or who are addicted to it may experience longer-term health effects, such as sexual impotence, liver damage, stomach problems, and damage to the heart. They may also have vitamin deficiencies and impaired immune systems, leaving susceptible to a wide variety of illnesses.

People Who Should Not Drink Alcohol. Some individuals should not drink any alcohol. For example, women who are pregnant or considering becoming pregnant should not drink because alcohol can affect a fetus, causing health impairments such as FETAL ALCOHOL SYNDROME (FAS). Others who should refrain from drinking include those addicted to alcohol, people with health problems such as ulcers that would be worsened by drinking, and people who are taking medications that would interact with alcohol. [*See also* ALCOHOL ADDICTION; ALCOHOL, DRUG/MEDICATION INTERACTIONS WITH; DRIVING WHILE INTOXICATED OR DRUG IMPAIRED.]

ALCOHOL ABUSE Excessive consumption of alcoholic beverages that leads to INTOXICATION or to ALCOHOL ADDICTION. Even if a person who abuses ALCOHOL does not become addicted, many serious consequences can result from excessive drinking, such as car crashes and various health problems.

According to the Substance Abuse and Mental Health Services Administration (SAMHSA), about 5.6 million people have an alcohol-abuse problem in the United States. Another 8 million people, or 10 percent of all drinkers, meet the criteria for ALCO-

HOLISM, which is characterized by a psychological need for and a physical ADDICTION to alcohol.

Criteria for Alcohol Abuse. According to the National Institute on Alcohol Abuse and Alcoholism (NIAAA), alcohol abuse is a drinking pattern accompanied by at least one of the following situations over the course of one year:

- Failing to perform responsibilities at work, school, or home
- Drinking while operating a car or machinery
- Being arrested for alcohol-related problems, such as drunk driving or assaulting someone while drunk
- Drinking despite relationship problems caused by or worsened with alcohol

Teenagers and Drinking. Although most adolescents do not drink, a significant number (about 30 percent) begin drinking between ages 12 and 17. Studies show that when adolescents start drinking at age 14 or younger, this early alcohol abuse will lead to an addiction to alcohol for about 40 percent of them. This sharply contrasts with those who delay drinking until age 21 or later: 10 percent of later drinkers develop a problem with alcoholism.

Most adolescents say that they consume alcohol to get along with others or because others are drinking, not because of a preference for the taste of alcohol. Many also wish to see what effect alcohol will have on them if they have never drunk it before. The desire for social approval starts young. In a study of children in the fourth through sixth grades 40 percent said that they would consume alcohol in order to fit in with the group or to seem older.

Sometimes the intense desire for social approval from friends and peers leads young people to engage in BINGE DRINKING, which is excessive and rapid drinking for at least one day in the past month. Adolescents and young adults may be pressured into such drinking by peers, who urge them on and call them names if they refrain from heavy drinking. Yet binge drinking can lead to death from ALCOHOL POISONING.

Primary Groups of People Who Drink. There are distinct patterns among people most likely to abuse alcohol based on such factors as gender, race, and educational status. For example, males are more likely to abuse alcohol than females. In a study of high school seniors 39 percent of the boys said they consumed five or more drinks at one time in the past 30 days, compared to 29 percent of the girls. Among adults men are about four times more likely to be heavy drinkers than women.

Alcohol abuse also varies among racial groups, with Hispanics and Caucasians the heaviest consumers of alcohol according to the *1998 National Household Survey on Drug Abuse.* Among adoles-

Percent Reporting Heavy Alcohol Use, by Race and Age	
White	
All Ages	**Ages 12–17**
5.8	3.5
Hispanic	
All Ages	**Ages 12–17**
6.2	2.3
African American	
All Ages	**Ages 12–17**
4.7	0.7

[Source: *National Household Survey on Drug Abuse: Population Estimates 1998 and 1999*, 1999.]

cent heavy drinkers ages 12–17 whites were the greatest consumers of alcohol, followed by Hispanics. Fewer than 1 percent of
black teens are heavy drinkers. Native Americans also have a high
rate of alcohol abuse. In a study of car crash deaths caused by alcohol, American Indians and Alaska Natives had a rate of 19.2
crashes per 100,000 in 1995. This was triple the rate for blacks
(6.4) and whites (6.0).

Even whether a person graduated from high school or not is a
factor in later alcohol abuse. Among adults those who did not
graduate from high school had the highest rate of heavy drinking
(7.5 percent). High school graduates (6.3 percent) fared about the
same as those with some college (6.6 percent). College graduates
had the lowest rate of heavy drinking, at 4 percent.

Health Consequences of Alcohol Abuse. Long-term alcohol
abuse can create many medical problems, such as *high blood pressure* and *coronary heart disease* (see Volume 8). Alcoholics are
also at risk for various CANCERS, CIRRHOSIS of the liver, HEPATITIS,
and PSYCHOSIS. When people have both cirrhosis and hepatitis,
their outlook is very grim, and most people with these combined
diseases die within one to four years. Some studies indicate that
women who are heavy drinkers have a greater risk of developing
breast cancer (see Volume 8).

Link to Smoking and Drugs. Adolescents who abuse alcohol are
much more likely than nondrinkers to smoke or abuse drugs. In a
study of alcohol use among adolescents, reported by the Substance
Abuse and Mental Health Services Administration (SAMHSA) in
2000, researchers found that the more adolescent alcohol users
drank, the higher the probability that they also used ILLEGAL
DRUGS or smoked cigarettes.

The study divided teenagers into four groups: (1) nondrinkers, (2) drinkers who had fewer than four drinks at a time, (3) binge drinkers, who had five or more drinks on one to four occasions, and (4) heavy drinkers who drank five or more drinks over five times in the past month. The differences between the groups were startling. For example, only about 3 percent of the nondrinkers had used illegal drugs, compared to 53 percent of the heavy drinkers. Drinking was also associated with smoking, and heavier drinkers had a higher risk of smoking cigarettes. The study suggests that avoiding smoking will not only eliminate the health consequences associated with it, but also avoid the link of smoking to alcohol and drug abuse.

Crime and Alcohol Abuse. Excessive alcohol consumption is linked to crime, and studies indicate that in one of every four crimes, the perpetrator was drinking before committing the crime. One study showed that offenders were drinking in 15 percent of robberies, 26 percent of aggravated or simple *assaults* (see Volume 5), and 37 percent of *rapes* and *sexual assaults* (see Volume 5).

Other Consequences of Alcohol Abuse. People who drink to excess may commit acts of sexual or physical abuse or become victims of abuse themselves. Because people's normal inhibitions disappear when they are intoxicated, they may also engage in *unprotected sex* (see Volume 3). The consequences may extend further. Unsafe sex could lead to an *unintended pregnancy* (see Volume 3) or to infections or other *sexually transmitted diseases (STDs)* (see Volume 7). When a woman abuses alcohol during pregnancy, her child is at risk for FETAL ALCOHOL SYNDROME (FAS), a serious problem with lifelong consequences. Alcohol abuse is also linked to *homicide, suicide* (see Volume 5), and CHILD ABUSE, as well as injuries or death from falls, drowning, and fires.

Treating Alcohol Abuse. A variety of methods may help people overcome their alcohol problem, whether they persistently abuse alcohol or are at risk for or already have alcoholism. SUPPORT GROUPS, ALCOHOL AND DRUG REHABILITATION PROGRAMS, and medications may help individuals with a continuing alcohol abuse problem. Therapists can help the individuals gain insight and better control over their problem.

Many experts recommend that anyone with an alcohol-abuse problem should practice complete ABSTINENCE from alcohol. They advise alcohol abusers to obtain medical help and attend support-group meetings such as those held by ALCOHOLICS ANONYMOUS (AA) or other self-help organizations. Family members and friends can help individuals by supporting their efforts to abstain from alcohol and not urging them to consume it in social situations. For a person with a continuing problem with alcohol, even just one drink is too much.

Some experts believe that people who abuse alcohol may be trying to self-medicate with alcohol in the hopes of blotting out an underlying problem with *depression* or *anxiety* (see Volume 2). Prescribed medications, such as antidepressants to treat severe depression, might help these people end their reliance on alcohol. However, experts disagree on whether medications can help.

ALCOHOL ADDICTION Physical and psychological need for ALCOHOL that is also known as ALCOHOLISM. When those addicted to alcohol do not consume it, they may experience symptoms of WITHDRAWAL, such as HALLUCINATIONS, shakiness, and convulsions. Long-term alcohol ADDICTION can lead to health problems such as CIRRHOSIS of the liver, HEPATITIS, CANCERS, and even severe psychological problems such as PSYCHOSIS.

There are a number of behaviors that can indicate an alcohol addiction. For example, alcoholics do not need a social occasion to drink and frequently drink alone. In fact, they may drink when they wake up in the morning, a strong indicator of alcohol addiction. Employers, coworkers, or schoolteachers may note indications of possible alcoholism. For example, if an individual is often absent from work or school, especially on Mondays (possibly after a weekend of drinking), this may be an indication of possible alcohol addiction or DRUG ABUSE. Also, if a person's work on the job or in school has declined dramatically and the individual is suddenly not getting along with coworkers or other students, this is another sign of a problem that may be either alcohol- or drug-related.

Alcohol addiction has a profound impact on the society as well as on the individual. According to the National Institute on Alcohol Abuse and Alcoholism, over half of all adults in the United States have a close family member who is now or has been addicted to alcohol. Alcohol addiction is linked to violence. In a study of alcoholic men in treatment half of them had been violent with their intimate partners within the year before their treatment for alcoholism began. Their levels of violence decreased with successful treatment.

ALCOHOL ADDICTION, CAUSES OF The factors that lead to ALCOHOL ADDICTION, or ALCOHOLISM. Experts have debated for years why people become addicted to ALCOHOL. In the past many people believed that the primary or sole cause of alcoholism was either a weak moral character or bad upbringing, with parents

Alcohol Dependence in the U.S., 1998

Problems in the Past Year Attributed to Alcohol Use Total Population	12–17	18–25	26–34	35+	Total
WANTED OR TRIED TO CUT DOWN BUT COULD NOT	4.1	7.2	5.0	3.1	4.1
BUILT UP TOLERANCE	6.4	18.2	8.7	4.3	7.0
USED ALCOHOL MORE THAN INTENDED	6.5	15.9	10.2	5.6	7.7
REDUCED IMPORTANT ACTIVITIES	2.0	5.1	2.5	1.3	2.0
CAUSED PSYCHOLOGICAL PROBLEMS	3.2	5.7	3.1	1.8	2.6
CAUSED HEALTH PROBLEMS	1.5	2.9	1.5	1.2	1.5
Any Alcohol Use in Past Year					
WANTED OR TRIED TO CUT DOWN BUT COULD NOT	12.9	9.7	6.8	4.9	6.4
BUILT UP TOLERANCE	20.0	24.5	11.7	6.6	10.9
USED ALCOHOL MORE THAN INTENDED	20.3	21.5	13.7	8.7	12.1
REDUCED IMPORTANT ACTIVITIES	6.3	6.9	3.4	2.0	3.2
CAUSED PSYCHOLOGICAL PROBLEMS	10.0	7.7	4.2	2.7	4.1
CAUSED HEALTH PROBLEMS	4.6	3.9	2.0	1.9	2.3
Binge Drinkers*					
WANTED OR TRIED TO CUT DOWN BUT COULD NOT	31.9	23.0	23.1	25.4	24.6
BUILT UP TOLERANCE	47.3	59.6	39.7	31.3	42.3
USED ALCOHOL MORE THAN INTENDED	54.8	53.9	45.6	38.3	45.3
REDUCED IMPORTANT ACTIVITIES	18.7	18.3	13.0	11.5	14.2
CAUSED PSYCHOLOGICAL PROBLEMS	23.9	19.6	18.4	15.2	17.6
CAUSED HEALTH PROBLEMS	11.5	11.1	10.7	10.0	10.9

*Binge drinkers are those who had five or more drinks on each of five or more occasions in the past 30 days

[Source: SAMHSA, *National Household Survey on Drug Abuse*, 1998.]

who failed to set a good example or who ignored their children. Today most experts recognize alcoholism as a disease that can be controlled with the help of physicians, family members, medications, and groups such as ALCOHOLICS ANONYMOUS (AA).

Environmental factors may play a role in alcohol addiction. For example, a person is more likely to become addicted if peers, parents, or siblings are also addicted to alcohol. There is also evidence of a genetic factor that may cause some people who start drinking to become alcoholics, while others never have this problem.

Some people believe that individuals with alcoholism often have underlying emotional problems, such as severe *depression* or *anxiety disorders* (see Volume 2), which contribute to their addiction. In their desire to rid themselves of the pain of these problems the individuals may abuse alcohol as a form of self-medication.

It is also possible that alcohol addiction may stem from a combination of factors. For example, a child may grow up in an unhappy environment with unloving or abusive parents. If that individual later engages in BINGE DRINKING, the heavy drinking could trigger an underlying genetic predisposition to addiction. It is very difficult to determine any single factor that may lead a person to becoming an alcoholic.

ALCOHOL ADDICTION, MEDICATIONS FOR See ADDICTION, MEDICATIONS FOR; ALCOHOL ADDICTION.

ALCOHOL ADVERTISING See ADVERTISING AND MEDIA.

ALCOHOL AND DRUG COUNSELING Assistance provided by a psychiatrist, psychologist, social worker, or therapist that enables a person to work on overcoming an ADDICTION to ALCOHOL or DRUGS. Counseling may entail meeting alone with a counselor or attending group meetings with others who have a drug or alcohol problem.

Individual counseling assists addicts by addressing not only the current alcohol or drug problems but also other issues in addicts' lives, such as family or work problems. The counselor may help addicts learn ways to deal with stressful problems in life so that once they are no longer addicted, they will be less likely to lapse into using drugs, alcohol, or tobacco as a way to cope with such problems.

Counselors also help addicts learn what types of actions seem to trigger the use of drugs or alcohol. Perhaps, for example, an individual always uses the substance after sex, at meal times, or on other specific occasions. Since recovering addicts will still want to have sex and need to eat, they must learn to associate other behaviors with these actions and to substitute these for using alcohol or drugs.

Group counseling is generally conducted with other individuals who have similar types of problem with either drugs or alcohol. Counselors often like to work with the families of alcohol or drug addicts to help them learn about more effective methods of coping with the problems that are caused by the disease.

Counseling alone may not be effective enough to overcome drug or alcohol addiction. Individuals may also need medications to combat their addiction. Regular follow-ups with counselors are also recommended, as well as participation in such self-help groups as ALCOHOLICS ANONYMOUS (AA).

ALCOHOL AND DRUG REHABILITATION PROGRAMS

Special programs to help people recover from addictions to ALCOHOL or DRUGS. Some programs are *residential*, which means that addicts live at a treatment center during the course of rehabilitation. Other programs offer *outpatient treatment*—addicts live at their own homes and go to a clinic or treatment center during the day for intensive therapy or counseling. Some alcohol and drug rehabilitation programs offer a combination of residential and outpatient therapy.

Most experts believe that residential programs are more effective at treating ADDICTION because all outside distractions are eliminated, and the addict is forced to concentrate on the program. A residential program provides 24-hour treatment. Experts report that drug abusers need at least 90 days of treatment. However, there are also short-term residential treatment programs (3–6 weeks), which are usually offered in a hospital and are then followed by therapy in a clinic.

Because residential treatment is extremely costly, at least two-thirds of all addicts are treated in outpatient programs. One key element of success in treating addiction appears to be follow-up or aftercare. In a study that compared alcoholics who had received outpatient treatment to those who had received aftercare after residential treatment or outpatient treatment, those who received the aftercare did the best. Twenty percent of the outpatient group was still practicing ABSTINENCE a year after treatment, compared to 35 percent of the aftercare group.

Steps to Rehabilitation. The first step in rehabilitation is usually DETOXIFICATION, a process in which the individual is taken off drugs or alcohol. He or she may need residential care during this phase for medical reasons, because WITHDRAWAL symptoms may be moderate to severe.

Detoxification is followed by the *recovery* process, during which addicts learn more about addiction in general as well as their own addiction problem. They also learn what they can expect as they recover. Counseling is very important at this stage, when the addict is most likely to pay close attention. Counselors teach addicted individuals techniques on how to utilize their strengths when they return home. Counselors also help addicted people realize that former friends and associates may have caused or contributed to the abuse problem because they too were addicted. As a result, addicts may be forced to give up certain friendships.

After the recovery period individuals return to society. Now, former alcohol or drug abusers must be very vigilant because it is after they return to their daily lives that they are most likely to abuse the substance again. If individuals can get past the three to six months after recovery, then they often have a good chance at maintaining abstinence from alcohol or drugs. However, most people continue to need SUPPORT GROUPS such as ALCOHOLICS ANONYMOUS (AA) to provide the motivation to keep them sober or drug free.

Problems and Challenges. One problem with some rehabilitation programs is that they concentrate on either drug or alcohol abuse but not both. Yet many people are addicted to both of these substances at the same time. A lesser problem, which experts are debating today, is whether residential programs should also help individuals quit smoking. Some experts say that it is too difficult to quit smoking when a person is also trying to stop drinking or taking drugs. Others argue that smoking is another addiction, and all addictions should be dealt with together, since smokers are more likely to be drinkers or drug takers.

ALCOHOL AND DRUGS, MALNUTRITION AND

Severely inadequate intake of nutrients as a result of abuse of ALCOHOL or DRUGS. People addicted to drugs or alcohol may become so obsessed with getting and using the substance that they ignore normal behaviors, including eating. As a result, they may not consume enough nutrients to maintain normal health, and this can lead to malnutrition.

Among alcoholics in particular, malnutrition can cause a worsening of existing liver diseases, such as HEPATITIS or CIRRHOSIS, that were initially caused by ALCOHOL ABUSE. Because a heavy consumption of alcohol can impair the process by which the body uses vitamins, alcoholics may also have vitamin deficiencies that may cause or contribute to the accelerated development of malnutrition.

One factor that contributes to the development of malnutrition among drug users is the fact that heavy drug use may impair the senses of taste and smell. As a result, food becomes unappetizing, and people addicted to drugs may thus have poor appetites. Abuse of COCAINE or AMPHETAMINES are most likely to lead to disinterest in eating, although other drugs may have the same effect.

ALCOHOL AND DRUGS, MOOD AND

The impact of ALCOHOL or DRUGS on the user's emotional state. Many people abuse alcohol or drugs because they believe that their mood will be dramatically heightened, and they will experience **euphoria** or other pleasurable feelings.

Although drugs or alcohol do change the mood of users, the direction of the change is usually beyond their control. People who use drugs or alcohol in order to attain a state of euphoria may just as easily find themselves becoming depressed, irritable, or aggressive and angry, depending on the drug, how much they took, and how long they have been using the substance.

Many people mistakenly believe that alcohol will make them feel happier. However, alcohol is actually a DEPRESSANT. It has a sedating effect and affects people in different ways. While drinking alcohol may make some individuals feel more relaxed and less tense, others who are intoxicated become sleepy and compliant. Still others may become irritable, angry, and mean.

Many legal and ILLEGAL DRUGS affect a person's mood, providing a temporary **rush**, or feeling of euphoria. Drugs may also greatly increase aggression and irritability. Abuse of some drugs such as COCAINE or ANABOLIC STEROIDS may cause serious psychological problems such as **paranoia**.

ALCOHOL AND DRUGS, SEX AND

Sexual actions and behaviors linked to the use of ALCOHOL or DRUGS. Some people believe that using alcohol or drugs will improve their sexual performance and satisfaction as well as those of their partner. However, ALCOHOL ABUSE or DRUG ABUSE often has the direct opposite effect.

When abusing alcohol or drugs, men may lose the ability to get and keep an erection or have an orgasm. Alcoholic men may have shrunken testicles. The use of AMPHETAMINES or COCAINE can make orgasm impossible for both men and women and can cause them to lose all sexual desire. HEROIN addicts often have impaired sexual drives and abilities.

Alcohol and drug abuse are also linked to risky sexual behaviors. People who are drugged or intoxicated are much less likely to use *condoms* during intercourse, increasing the risk of infection from HIV or other *sexually transmitted diseases (STDs)* such as *syphilis, gonorrhea,* or *herpes* (see Volume 7). Women who use alcohol and drugs are more likely to have *unintended pregnancies*

Keywords

euphoria an exaggerated feeling of well-being that has no basis in reality
paranoia irrational belief that others are out to harm you, a feature of some mental illnesses
rush a sudden feeling of intense euphoria brought on by the use of certain drugs

(see Volume 3). Moreover, studies show that adolescents and college students whose inhibitions have been impaired by alcohol or drugs are much more likely to engage in *unprotected sex* (see Volume 3).

ALCOHOL AND HEALTH PROBLEMS Medical problems caused by ALCOHOL ABUSE or ALCOHOL ADDICTION. Alcohol consumption can affect virtually every system of the body, from the digestive system to the cardiovascular system (which includes the heart and the bloodstream), to the central nervous system. Thus, when a person is a heavy or chronic alcohol user, the long-term health consequences can be very severe.

The Brain. Studies indicate that many people who are alcoholics have deteriorated brain function. The most extreme example is known as Korsakoff's syndrome, in which the person forgets events immediately after they happen. As a result, a person with this syndrome can only remember things from the distant past.

People with ALCOHOLISM may also experience ALCOHOLIC BLACKOUTS. These are periods of INTOXICATION during which a person may walk about and talk to others but later have no memory of these events whatsoever. Alcoholism can also cause brain shrinkage and early death of nerve cells in the brain. The most commonly affected area is the frontal part of the brain, in the area that enables a person to make plans and carry them out.

Alcoholics sometimes have a thiamin (Vitamin B_1) deficiency due to both poor nutrition and damage to the gastrointestinal tract that prevents normal absorption of the vitamin. This deficiency can cause massive damage to the part of the brain called the *cerebral cortex*, often resulting in memory loss as well as an overall difficulty in thinking.

The Liver. CIRRHOSIS of the liver is a common problem associated with alcohol abuse. At least 2 million Americans have some form of alcoholic liver disease, ranging from the early to later stages of cirrhosis. Heavy consumers of alcohol are also at risk for developing alcoholic HEPATITIS, an inflammation of the liver caused by excessive drinking (and a different disease from viral hepatitis). Treatment for alcoholic hepatitis is aimed at reducing the inflammation of the liver.

The Cardiovascular System. Chronic heavy drinking can cause the heart to enlarge. It may also decrease the heart's ability to contract, a condition called *alcoholic cardiopathy*. One symptom of this condition is shortness of breath. Alcoholism can cause other forms of heart disease as well. The most serious risk is a

Fact or Folklore?

Folklore It takes years of drinking before alcohol abuse affects the brain.

Recent studies indicate that even teenagers may suffer brain damage from heavy drinking. Researchers at the National Institute on Alcohol Abuse and Alcoholism (NIAAA) released findings in 2000 on 33 adolescents ages 15–16. All were heavy drinkers who were not dependent on other DRUGS. The researchers found significant differences between the performances of the alcoholic teenagers and a group of non-alcoholic teens on tests of learning, memory, language skills, problem solving, and attention. The researchers concluded that ALCOHOL can have quite different toxic effects on adolescent brains than on those of adults.

heart attack. Heavy drinking can also lead to irregular heart rhythms, and such *arrhythmias* (see Volume 8) can cause sudden death.

Regular heavy consumption of alcohol also contributes to *high blood pressure* (see Volume 8), also known as *hypertension*. In studies of men who consumed 2–6 drinks per day, their high blood pressure dropped significantly after abstaining from alcohol. High blood pressure is a major risk factor in both heart attack and *stroke* (see Volume 8).

The Bones. Researchers have learned that alcoholism is also linked to an increased risk of *osteoporosis* (see Volume 8). In this disorder the bones lose calcium and become porous and fragile. Osteoporosis is generally found in older people, particularly women, but for reasons still unclear, alcohol causes or contributes to this condition.

According to experts, heavy alcohol use can damage the developing bones of adolescents, leading to a higher risk of osteoporosis as adults. Bones normally grow at a rapid pace during adolescence. With alcoholic adolescents, however, the bones may not reach their full potential. Teenagers who abuse alcohol could thus be creating the possibility for weak or deformed bones in later adult life. If diagnosed in time, osteoporosis can be treated with medications, but the medicines also have side effects, such as stomach upset.

The Circulatory System. Another system in the body that is harmed by heavy alcohol use is the circulatory system, particularly the healthy production of red and white blood cells. Alcohol abuse impairs the body's ability to fight off infections by harming the production of white blood cells. This weakens the *immune system* (see Volume 7) and increases the risk of diseases such as *pneumonia* and *tuberculosis* (see Volume 8). Some experts believe that alcoholics are also more susceptible to contracting *HIV infections* (see Volume 7). People who are alcoholics also often have damaged red blood cells, although experts disagree on why and how this happens. The result, however, is that they may develop *anemia* (see Volume 8).

Another serious problem for the circulatory system caused by excessive alcohol consumption is its effect on the blood clotting process, making clots more likely to form. If a clot in a blood vessel blocks the blood flow to the brain, it can cause a stroke. People who are heavy alcohol abusers are thus at greater risk of suffering from strokes, and many die from them.

The Male Reproductive System. Studies have shown that heavy alcohol consumption causes a decreased production of the male

---

VICTIMS OF DISEASES LINKED TO ALCOHOLISM

The health problems associated with alcoholism strike some races harder than others. For example, researchers report that deaths from CIRRHOSIS of the liver are most frequent among American Indians/ Alaska Natives, who suffer a very high rate of 25.9 deaths per 100,000 individuals. This is nearly three times greater than the next closest rate of 9.9 per 100,000 people, suffered by African Americans.

The rate of whites with cirrhosis is nearly the same as that for African Americans—9.4 per 100,000 individuals. Asian/Pacific Islanders are the least affected from this ailment, with a rate of only 3.5 deaths per 100,000. They also are least likely to be alcoholics.

Men are more likely to suffer health problems as a result of alcoholism than women. The primary reason for this is that men are more likely than women to be alcoholic.

hormone testosterone and can even shrink the testes. As many as 75 percent of men with advanced alcoholic cirrhosis have shrunken testicles. Low levels of testosterone among alcoholic men also contribute to a greater risk for impotence and infertility. Moreover, the lower levels of testosterone in alcoholic men may cause them to develop more feminine features, such as less facial and chest hair and breast enlargement (a condition known as *gynemastia*).

The Female Reproductive System. Alcoholic women may also develop problems with their reproductive systems. Studies have shown that women who consume more than three drinks a day have a greater risk of having problems with ovulation, the release of an egg cell, which, when combined with sperm, results in a fertilized egg and eventually a fetus. Heavy alcohol abuse can delay ovulation or prevent it from occurring. Without ovulation **pregnancy** (see Volume 3) cannot occur, so women alcoholics may be infertile.

Heavy female drinkers are also at risk for menstrual problems, and some studies indicate that alcoholic women have an increased risk of developing **breast cancer** (see Volume 8).

Of alcoholic women who have babies, many have difficulty with breast-feeding. Alcohol impedes the release of the hormone prolactin, which is normally stimulated by the infant's suckling. The result is that the baby cannot obtain enough nutrition because of an inadequate amount of breast milk. Infants born to women who abused alcohol during pregnancy are also at high risk for FETAL ALCOHOL SYNDROME (FAS), which includes physical and mental impairments.

The Pancreas. The pancreas is an organ of the body that produces certain hormones and digestive juices. Chronic heavy drinking can lead to a severe condition called *alcoholic pancreatitis*, which is usually characterized by severe abdominal pain and vomiting. Alcoholic men in their forties are most at risk for this serious disease. In mild cases alcoholic pancreatitis can be treated, but in severe cases the person becomes very sick, and about 30 percent die. A person with a sudden and severe attack of alcoholic pancreatitis usually must have intravenous fluids in the hospital along with complete bed rest and pain medication. In the case of chronic pancreatitis ABSTINENCE from alcohol will decrease pain and cut back on the number of severe attacks. Medications also may help.

The Gastrointestinal System. Chronic alcohol abuse can harm the esophagus (the food tube that leads to the stomach), causing severe acid reflux, or heartburn. Chronic acid reflux can lead to a precancerous condition called *Barrett's esophagus*.

Mallory-Weiss syndrome, another digestive disorder suffered by many alcoholics, causes heavy internal bleeding in the area where the esophagus joins the stomach. In about half of patients with this disorder the cause was pressure resulting from repeated episodes of vomiting after very heavy drinking.

Alcohol abuse also contributes to the development of CANCERS in the gastrointestinal system, such as esophageal cancer and rectal cancer. When drinkers also smoke, the risk can be up to 45 times greater than the risk for the person who does not drink or smoke.

The Teeth and Mouth. Alcoholics have a higher risk of contracting ORAL CANCER than nonalcoholics. When they also smoke, the risk is even greater. Alcohol abuse also increases the risk of tooth decay, gum disease, and of losing teeth.

ALCOHOL AND MENTAL HEALTH See Volume 2.

ALCOHOL AND VIOLENCE
The association of the use of alcohol with violent acts. Alcohol is implicated in many acts of violence, ranging from *assault* (see Volume 5) to CHILD ABUSE or DOMESTIC VIOLENCE AND ABUSE all the way to *homicide* (see Volume 5). Of about 11 million victims of violent crime each year, 2.7 million reported that the offender had been drinking alcohol before committing the crime.

Research indicates that women who are substance abusers are more likely to be attacked than other women. For example, in one study of women receiving treatment for ALCOHOLISM, 73 percent had a prior history of being a victim of *rape* (see Volume 5) or assault. Experts debate why alcoholic women are more likely to become victims of violence and whether alcoholism is a cause or an effect. It is unknown whether most such women may have turned to alcohol as a result of an attack or if they were more vulnerable to attack *because* they were frequently intoxicated. What is clear, however, is that alcohol abuse and violence go together. Similar results have been found among women who abuse DRUGS.

ALCOHOL AND WITHDRAWAL See ALCOHOL ADDICTION; WITHDRAWAL.

ALCOHOL, DRUG/MEDICATION INTERACTIONS WITH
The effects of combining the use of ALCOHOL, DRUGS, and medications. The combined effect on the body of taking drugs or medications along with alcohol may be one of decreased or increased action, or it may change how the medication acts in some other way. Drinking even a small amount of alcohol can change how a drug affects the body. In the most extreme cases the drug-alcohol interaction could cause coma or death.

Interactions between Alcohol and Varioius Classes of Medications

Drug Class	Type of Interaction
ANALGESICS (PAIN RELIEF)	ASPIRIN LEADS TO FASTER ALCOHOL ABSORPTION IN SMALL INTESTINE. USE OF ALCOHOL WITH ACETAMINOPHEN (TYLENOL) INCREASES POTENTIAL FOR LIVER DAMAGE
ANTIBIOTICS (MICROBIAL INFECTION)	ERYTHROMYCIN MAY LEAD TO FASTER ALCOHOL ABSORPTION IN SMALL INTESTINE
ANTICONVULSANTS (SEIZURE DISORDERS)	CHRONIC ALCOHOL CONSUMPTION INDUCES BREAK DOWN OF THE ANTI-CONVULSANT DRUG DILANTIN
ANTIHISTAMINES (ALLERGIES, COLDS)	ALCOHOL ENHANCES EFFECTS OF ANTI-HISTAMINES ON THE CENTRAL NERVOUS SYSTEM, INCREASING DROWSINESS AND SEDATION AND DECREASING MOTOR SKILLS. INTERACTION OF ALCOHOL AND ANTIHISTAMINES IS MORE MARKED IN PEOPLE OVER AGE 65
BARBITURATES	CHRONIC ALCOHOL USE INCREASES BARBITURATE METABOLISM AND ENHANCES SEDATING AND HYPNOTIC EFFECTS OF BARBITURATES
MUSCLE RELAXANTS	ALCOHOL WORSENS IMPAIRMENT OF PHYSICAL ABILITIES (SUCH AS DRIVING) AND INCREASES SEDATION
OPIOIDS (PAIN RELIEF)	ALCOHOL CAUSES MORE DROWSINESS AND FURTHER DECREASES MOTOR SKILLS
SEDATIVES AND HYPNOTICS	ALCOHOL INHIBITS METABOLISM OF THESE DRUGS, PRODUCING A DEPRESSANT EFFECT OF SLEEPINESS, DISORIENTATION, AND CONFUSION
SOME ANTIDEPRESSANTS (DEPRESSION)	ALCOHOL INCREASES RISK OF SEDATION AND RISK OF SUDDEN DROP IN BLOOD PRESSURE WHEN PERSON STANDS UP
HERBAL MEDICATIONS (SLEEP AIDS)	ALCOHOL MAY INCREASE DROWSINESS ASSOCIATED WITH THESE PREPARATIONS

[Source: National Institute on Drug Abuse, *Alcohol Research: Health*, 23, 1, 1999.]

Alcohol and Medication Interactions. Many different categories of medications interact with alcohol, including BARBITURATES, muscle relaxants, ANTIBIOTICS, antidepressants, pain medications, OPIATES, and antihistamines. Many over-the-counter medications and herbal remedies also interact with alcohol.

Just because a product is found in a drugstore or a health food store or is labeled "natural" does not mean that it is always safe to take with alcohol. For example, chamomile, echinacea, or valerian are all herbal remedies for insomnia that are thought to produce drowsiness. But if any of these drugs are combined with alcohol, the drowsiness is increased even further.

Some medications cause a severe reaction when mingled with alcohol and may cause nausea, vomiting, flushing (reddening of the skin), and sweating. These effects are similar to the response that the body has to taking ANTABUSE, a drug given to alcoholics to stop them from drinking. Among the medications that can cause such reactions are some diabetes medications, cardiac medicines, and many antibiotics. Alcohol taken with some pain relievers such as ibuprofen can cause gastrointestinal bleeding.

Alcohol and Illegal Drugs. It is often dangerous to consume alcohol and ILLEGAL DRUGS at the same time. People who use both substances risk falling victim to various injuries and death. If the illegal drug is a depressant, abusers also risk oversedation and, in the worst case, brain damage leading to coma or death. With the use of stimulants they risk causing a heart attack or *stroke* (see Volume 8).

ALCOHOL EXPERIMENTATION

Trying ALCOHOL to test its effects. Adolescents and even children may experiment with alcohol use primarily because they are urged to do so by peers or because they are curious about the effect it may have on them. However, even a one-time use of alcohol can be dangerous, particularly if the intoxicated person decides to drive a car or operate any heavy or dangerous equipment. If the experimentation involves BINGE DRINKING, it could lead to a serious and potentially fatal condition known as ALCOHOL POISONING.

Some parents allow their underage children to drink at home under their supervision in the belief that this practice will prevent their children from drinking outside the home. However, studies have shown that the reverse is true. Children and adolescents who are allowed to drink at home are more likely to develop problems with ALCOHOL ABUSE. [*See also* PEER PRESSURE AND ADDICTION.]

ALCOHOLIC BLACKOUT

A state of amnesia (lack of memory) of all events that occur during a state of extreme intoxication. Victims of alcoholic blackouts are conscious and may have walked around and talked to others, but later they do not remember these actions at all. The alcoholic blackout is a sign of severe ALCOHOL ABUSE or ALCOHOLISM. The risk for this condition is increased when individuals use sedating DRUGS along with alcohol. Severe fatigue combined with heavy alcohol consumption may also increase the risk for an alcoholic blackout.

ALCOHOLICS ANONYMOUS (AA) An organization whose goal is to help people handle their ALCOHOL ADDICTION. Founded in 1935, Alcoholics Anonymous (AA) is an international organization with more than 1 million members in the United States in about 50,000 groups nationwide. There are an additional 770,000 members worldwide. The only requirement for membership in Alcoholics Anonymous is that the member wants to stop drinking. AA does not charge dues. About 98 percent of the members are over age 21, and about two-thirds are men.

AA is "anonymous" because members do not use their last names at meetings, and information discussed there is confidential. Meetings are designated as either open or closed, and every AA group has both types of meetings. Family members and guests may come to open meetings, but only alcoholics may attend closed meetings.

Anonymity is a very important concept to AA members and to the organization. AA believes that anonymity gives individuals the freedom to reveal information that would be hard to share otherwise, such as personal problems caused by ALCOHOL ABUSE. The principle of anonymity also lessens the fear a person might have that other members might tell nonmembers about what is said in meetings.

A basic strategy of AA is the TWELVE-STEP PROGRAM. The first step in this program is accepting one's own powerlessness over ALCOHOLISM. The second step is admitting that a greater power beyond oneself could restore sanity.

The other steps in the Twelve-Step Program are: deciding to give over one's will to God or a higher power (as understood by the individual); taking a hard look at oneself; admitting one's wrongs to the higher power, oneself, and another person; readying oneself to have the higher power remove character defects; asking the higher power to remove these defects; creating a list of people that one has harmed and being willing to atone for these harms; making amends to the people that one has harmed unless doing so would hurt them or others; continuing a personal analysis of oneself and freely admitting faults; praying and meditating; and carrying the message to others who are alcoholics. [*See also* AL-ANON; ALATEEN; SUPPORT GROUPS.]

ALCOHOLISM ADDICTION TO ALCOHOL. Alcoholism is a disease that can have serious health consequences for an individual. It is estimated that about 8 million people—10 percent of all drinkers—in the United States suffer from alcoholism.

According to the National Institute on Alcohol Abuse and Alcoholism (NIAAA), there are four symptoms of alcoholism. The first symptom is a need or craving for alcohol and a compulsion to drink. Second, alcoholics lose control over their drinking; and once they start to drink, they cannot have only one or two drinks but must drink to excess. Physical dependence is a third symptom of alcoholism. This means that if a person goes without alcohol, he or she will suffer from certain physical WITHDRAWAL symptoms, such as nausea, sweating, and shakiness, which are also among the symptoms of DELIRIUM TREMENS (DTs). These withdrawal symptoms only go away if the person has a drink. The fourth symptom of alcoholism is tolerance, which creates a physical need for greater amounts of alcohol than were required in the past.

There are many health problems associated with alcoholism, such as CIRRHOSIS of the liver, brain damage, infertility, *anemia* (see Volume 8), *osteoporosis* (see Volume 4), and diseases of the gastrointestinal system. [See also ALCOHOL AND HEALTH PROBLEMS; DEPENDENCE, PHYSICAL; TOLERANCE, PHYSICAL.]

ALCOHOLISM TREATMENT Methods to help treat those suffering from an ADDICTION TO ALCOHOL. In 1999 an estimated 2.3 million people in the United States received some form of treatment for ALCOHOLISM.

There are a variety of treatments that experts recommend for alcoholics. The most important first step in alcoholism treatment is for the alcoholic to recognize that there is a problem and be willing to accept help. When alcoholics are unwilling to accept help, sometimes friends or family members may intervene to try to convince or compel the person to accept some form of treatment. If an alcoholic has committed a crime, part of the sentence may require the person to complete alcoholism treatment, or it may be a condition for avoiding time in jail.

Some individuals combat alcoholism with the help of a psychiatrist or psychologist. Others seek the aid of such self-help groups as ALCOHOLICS ANONYMOUS (AA). Still others may need to enter a residential program for people who abuse alcohol. Another option, which may be used along with some of the other methods, is to use medication to curb the desire to drink.

Treatment with Professional Therapy. Many psychiatrists, psychologists, nurses, and social workers are involved in helping alcoholics overcome their addiction. These professionals may use

Keywords

behavior therapy form of psychotherapy that uses learning and conditioning techniques to change undesirable behavior
tolerance capacity of the body to endure or become less responsive to a substance with repeated use

a variety of methods to help their patients. One such method, known as **behavior therapy**, teaches alcoholics to challenge wrong ideas that they may have about the world and about themselves. A simple example of this therapy in action might be to challenge the idea, If I fail at something, then I am a bad person. The therapist would guide the patient to a more rational thought, such as, If I fail at something, I may not be skilled at that task, or I might need more practice at it. The therapist teaches alcoholics to challenge negative attitudes they may have about themselves or others.

The therapist might also teach relaxation techniques. For example, instead of habitually using alcohol as a way to deal with stress, alcoholics could learn how to relax tense muscle groups. A therapist might also ask individuals to imagine a placid scene that enables them to calm themselves.

Group therapy (see Volume 2) may also help the alcoholic. Led by a therapist, the group discusses problems and possible solutions. *Family therapy* (see Volume 2) is another form of treatment for alcoholics. In this type of therapy the therapist helps the family and the alcoholic learn better ways of coping with daily problems. Problem issues that were unknown or ignored by others are often brought out by family members during such sessions. For example, an alcoholic father may learn in a group therapy session that his son is ashamed to bring friends home because of his father's drunken behavior. This realization may lead to a resolve to continue treatment and stop drinking.

Alcoholics Anonymous. A self-help group that has helped millions deal with alcoholism, Alcoholics Anonymous (AA) offers people who abuse alcohol an opportunity to meet with other alcoholics and discuss problems. More importantly, it gives alcoholics a chance to meet others who have been severe alcohol abusers and yet managed to overcome the lure of alcohol.

Members of AA advocate complete ABSTINENCE from alcohol and are very firm in this belief. Some people believe that an alcoholic may learn to become a moderate or occasional drinker, but that view is not accepted by most experts or by Alcoholics Anonymous.

Residential Treatment. There are a variety of residential treatment centers that specialize in helping alcoholics become sober. They may provide individual and group therapy, discussion groups, medication, and other methods that have proven successful in the past.

In some cases before entering residential treatment alcoholics may need to enter a hospital so that they can be under medical supervision as they go through the physical and psychological effects of WITHDRAWAL from alcohol.

Studies have found that residential treatment of about a year is more successful in treating alcoholism than shorter-term treatment. Many people, however, cannot afford such a long period of treatment, nor are they willing to be away from their families for that long. In such cases they may be treated for several months. Whether addicts receive residential treatment or not, they will need follow-up, which may involve attending group or individual therapy sessions in a clinic or hospital setting.

Medications That Help. The primary medication used to treat alcoholism in the past was ANTABUSE. A person who takes this drug and then also drinks alcohol will experience severe vomiting. This treatment has had mixed results. Some experts believe that combining Antabuse with other medications may be effective, and studies are underway to test this idea.

Older antidepressant medications (such as desipramine or imipramine) have proven effective with some people who abuse alcohol. Newer antidepressants, such as Prozac (fluoxetine), also help some alcoholics. How can antidepressants help? The theory is that some alcohol abusers drink because they are severely depressed. According to this view, if the depression is gone, the need to drink will diminish or disappear.

Experts also use other medications in addition to Antabuse and antidepressants. ReVia (naltrexone) is a medication that has been used to treat alcohol abuse since the early 1990s. NALTREXONE blocks the pleasure centers of the brain from being stimulated by alcohol. Thus a person who takes naltrexone and then drinks will not have the pleasurable or euphoric feelings they felt in the past when consuming alcohol.

One problem with using medications is that they only work if taken as prescribed. Many people, however, have trouble remembering to take medicines, or they refuse to take them. Another problem with medications (other than Antabuse) is that the person may continue to drink and also take the drug, risking side effects.

ALCOHOL LAWS Laws that regulate the sale of alcoholic beverages, indicating who may sell them and under what conditions. Some states in the U.S. have a monopoly on the sale of alcohol, while others license only certain retailers to sell liquor. There are also laws to punish those convicted of ***drunk driving*** (see Volume 5).

All states prohibit the sale of alcohol to people under age 21. They also provide punishments for retailers who illegally sell alcohol to those who are under the legal age, as well as punishments for private citizens who buy alcohol for minors.

States also have laws relating to certain alcohol-based crimes. For example, drivers with BLOOD ALCOHOL LEVELS at or above a certain limit set by the state may be arrested. Repeat offenders caught DRIVING WHILE INTOXICATED OR DRUG IMPAIRED are usually subject to more severe penalties.

All states also have so-called ZERO TOLERANCE LAWS, which make it illegal for anyone under age 21 to drink and drive. Since about 1998 the states have set blood alcohol levels of between zero and 0.02 as unacceptable levels of INTOXICATION for individuals under age 21. Early indications suggest the zero tolerance laws have been somewhat successful in reducing the number drunk-driving fatalities among youth.

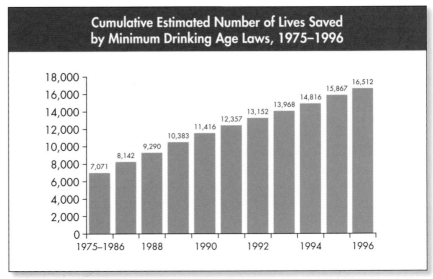

Cumulative Estimated Number of Lives Saved by Minimum Drinking Age Laws, 1975–1996

[Source: Substance Abuse and Mental Health Services Administration, *Impaired Driving among Youth: Trends and Tools for Prevention*, 1999.]

Keywords

diuretic substance that increases the volume of urine excreted form the kidneys
metabolize break down chemically within the body

ALCOHOL, METABOLISM OF The process by which the body breaks down and absorbs ALCOHOL. Once absorbed into the bloodstream, about 90 percent of alcohol is **metabolized** in the liver; the rest is metabolized in the stomach, kidney, and other tissues and then excreted in urine, sweat, and the breath.

Because the liver is responsible for metabolizing most of the alcohol consumed, it must work more than normal to accomplish this process. As a result, constant heavy abuse of alcohol can be quite damaging to the overworked liver. Long-term ALCOHOL ABUSE can lead to CIRRHOSIS of the liver or HEPATITIS. Studies of alcoholic adolescents have shown that liver damage can begin early.

ALCOHOL OVERDOSE An excessive consumption of ALCOHOL that results in INTOXICATION, sickness, unconsciousness, and, in rare cases, death. The *hangover* is a common condition resulting from a prior alcohol overdose. It is characterized by headache, nausea, fatigue, dizziness, thirst, stomach pain, increased sweating, and irritability.

The symptoms of a hangover generally start several hours after drinking ends. The aftereffects of the action of alcohol on the body are what cause a hangover. For example, excessive alcohol acts as a **diuretic**, making the kidneys pump out more fluid than was consumed. As a result, the person becomes dehydrated and extremely thirsty. Heavy drinking also irritates the stomach and can cause gastritis, an inflammation of the stomach lining.

For most people with hangovers the best treatment is rest, sleep, and plenty of fluids. Symptoms usually end within 8 to 24 hours. Bland foods such as crackers may help decrease nausea, while some medications may help relieve other hangover symptoms, such as antacids to relieve gastritis. Caffeine reportedly may also help, although studies have not proven that it works. It is important to note that caffeine will *not* work in ending intoxication early. The liver processes alcohol at a steady rate, and drinking coffee or other caffeine drinks, such as cola, will not speed up the metabolism of alcohol by the liver.

Some substances should be avoided by people with a hangover. For example, acetaminophen (Tylenol) should not be taken, because it can irritate the liver, which has already been irritated by the ALCOHOL ABUSE. A person with a hangover should also avoid consuming any additional quantities of alcohol.

ALCOHOL POISONING is a very dangerous and special case of an alcoholic overdose. It often results from BINGE DRINKING over a period that was too short to allow the body to absorb the toxic effects of massive quantities of alcohol. Alcohol poisoning can be fatal.

ALCOHOL POISONING A reaction to toxic levels of ALCOHOL in the blood caused by drinking extreme quantities over a very short period of time. Drinking an excessive amount of alcohol depresses the central nervous system, slowing blood pressure and breathing. In alcohol poisoning, BLOOD ALCOHOL LEVELS may be as high as 0.4 percent, which is more than four times the legal INTOXICATION limit in most states.

Alcohol poisoning is a medical crisis that can lead to death, either because a person chokes on his or her own vomit or because breathing slows down to the point where there is not enough oxygen to sustain life. BINGE DRINKING is a major cause of alcohol poisoning, and anyone who drinks large amounts of alcohol in a short period of time is at risk. Alcohol poisoning most commonly occurs among young people who are DRINKING IN COLLEGE, usually binge drinking.

There are several major indicators of possible alcohol poisoning. One sign is that the drunken person cannot be wakened by shaking or speaking very loudly to him or her. Another indicator is skin that is cold or clammy and perhaps pale or bluish in tone. If a person vomits without waking, this is another sign of alcohol poisoning. Erratic breathing, with ten or more seconds between breaths, is also a danger sign, as is very slow breathing of eight or fewer breaths per minute.

Anyone who finds a person who may be a victim of alcohol poisoning should call an ambulance immediately. In the meantime the victim should be turned on the side so that if vomiting occurs during unconsciousness, the person will not choke on the vomit. The victims should not be left alone, because they may change their position and then start choking to death.

ALTERNATIVE MEDICINE Methods and treatments that are not part of western, scientific medical practice. Many such treatments expose people to unregulated or unmonitored drugs, overly expensive and unproven regimens, and extreme or unbalanced dietary practices. All should be adopted only with great caution and considerable skepticism, since reactions to or problems with unknown substances may be difficult to treat.

Alternative therapies include a wide range of practices that people use to treat a variety of ills. They fall into three broad groups: (1) those that have scientific evidence proving they are effective, (2) those that have scientific evidence proving they are not effective, and (3) those that experts are unsure about because the approaches have not yet been adequately studied. The first group of practices includes such things as relaxation therapy (for stress), biofeedback (for pain control), *group therapy* (see Volume 2) (for psychological or emotional difficulties), hypnosis (for behavioral ills), *yoga* (see Volume 4) (for stress), and the drinking of cranberry juice (for urinary tract infections). *Relaxation therapy* and yoga involve the deliberate relaxing and tensing of muscles as well as *meditation* exercises (see Volume 2). Biofeedback is a method for mentally controlling some normal body processes (such as heart beat and blood pressure). Various relaxation therapies may be useful during pregnancy and labor. They have also been used to treat alcoholism. Group therapy involves interaction among people who share common psychological problems. Psychiatrists and psychologists use hypnosis to powerfully suggest certain behaviors to patients.

The vast majority of alternative medical therapies falls into groups 2 and 3. For example, the use of vitamin C supplements to prevent the common cold has been scientifically proven to be ineffective. Scientists have not conducted enough research to determine the effectiveness of drinking green tea or eating the herb ginseng.

Scientific investigation of alternative medicine therapies is controversial. Proponents of alternative medicine say that scientists are often reluctant to study therapies that are so different from conventional medical treatments, so scientific evidence is lacking. Others say that science cannot properly assess alternative therapies at all because they work in ways that are too difficult for scientists to study. Most medical scientists disagree with this view because they have successfully conducted numerous studies on alternative treatments and gained important information about their safety and effectiveness. They say that the best way to assess alternative approaches is to apply the same scientific methods used in all other areas of medicine.

The National Institutes of Health divides alternative practices into five major categories:

1. *Alternative Medical Systems.* These are complete systems of theory and practice that in many cases were devised independently of conventional scientific medicine. Often traditional parts of a culture, they encompass many kinds of treatment, including homeopathy, naturopathy, and acupuncture. In homeopathy, a person takes small doses of a remedy that in a healthy person would produce symptoms of the disease being treated. Naturopathy makes use of natural agents such as heat, cold, water, sunshine, and physical means such as manipulation of the body and electrical pulses.

Some addicts have found relief from addiction by use of acupuncture, a therapy in which tiny needles are placed at trigger points of the body by a trained practitioner. Since 1996 the Food and Drug Administration (FDA) has approved the use of acupuncture by licensed individuals. In 2000, scientists at Yale University reported success in treating addiction to COCAINE with auricular acupuncture, in which needles are placed in the outer ear. The researchers found that 55 percent of the subjects receiving this treatment were drug-free after eight weeks. Further studies are being conducted on this therapy.

2. *Mind-body Interventions.* These are techniques that attempt to affect the body's functions and symptoms by using the mind. These approaches include the use of meditation, hypnosis, dance, music, and prayer. The object is to achieve a certain mental state so that physical healing can begin. Hypnosis is an alternative remedy that has helped some people gain relief from their addictions, especially those who wish to give up smoking. When hypnotized, the person willingly enters a trancelike state and is given instructions that are intended to help them stop the addictive behavior. Patients can also be trained to perform self-hypnosis on themselves.

3. Biological-based Therapies. These practices are intended to directly affect the body's biological or chemical functions. In this group are therapies that involve eating herbs, certain foods, high-dose vitamins or minerals, and other naturally derived substances. Although there are few herbs proven to be effective in treating addiction, researchers at the National Center for Complementary and Alternative Medicine (NCCAM) are testing six Chinese herb extracts as a possible treatment for alcoholism. Kudzu, a vine that grows wild in the southeastern United States, is the primary plant being considered in this study. Researchers have successfully isolated several chemicals in kudzu that may be effective in treating ALCOHOLISM, although further testing is needed.

Some experts belive that drugs such as St.-John's-wort, also used for treating *depression* (see Volume 2), may be effective in helping people end addictions. However, there is no scientific proof that this herbal drug actually works.

4. Manipulative and Body-based Methods. These practices are intended to directly affect the body's biological or chemical functions. In this group are therapies that include relaxation, yoga, and biofeedback.

5. Energy Therapies. These methods are intended to manipulate energy fields that can affect the body, some of which have not been scientifically proven to exist. Some of the most common energy therapies are therapeutic touch, Reiki, Qi gong, and the unconventional use of electromagnetic fields. Each focuses on a different kind of alleged energy that flows from the body.

MORE SOURCES See www.nccam.nih.gov; www.quackwatch.com

AMPHETAMINES Stimulant drugs first introduced in the 1930s as over-the-counter medications to relieve nasal congestion or combat *sleep disorders* (see Volume 8). During World War II many soldiers used the amphetamines Dexedrine and Methedrine to stay alert on the battlefield.

Up until the mid-1960s amphetamines, which are STIMULANTS, were prescribed for many different purposes, such as for weight loss, to treat *depression* (see Volume 2), or to help athletes improve their performance. It soon became apparent, however, that some people were abusing the drugs, as evidenced by increased hyperactivity or disturbed behavior in those who used them.

In response to this abuse in 1965 the Food and Drug Administration (FDA) sharply limited the manufacture of amphetamines. After that decision illegal laboratories began producing amphetamines, primarily METHAMPHETAMINE, a drug that soon became widely abused. One illegal form of methamphetamine known as "crystal meth" can be smoked.

Amphetamines are still used legally today. For example, the drug Ritalin is sometimes prescribed for children and adults diagnosed with attention-deficit disorder, an emotional disorder of people who have problems with impulsive behavior, above-average difficulty with concentration, and sometimes hyperactivity. Amphetamines are also prescribed for narcolepsy, a rare disease that causes a person to fall asleep suddenly and uncontrollably. Amphetamines may be taken orally or injected, and the effect lasts from two to four hours.

When abused, amphetamines are used to achieve a feeling of euphoria, or a "high." Amphetamine users may also feel in complete control, although the reality is that they have far *less* control than normal when under the influence of these drugs.

Physical and Emotional Reactions. Amphetamines increase blood pressure and heart rate. The drugs may also cause increased sweating, lack of coordination, blurred vision, and even physical collapse. Individuals who take amphetamines may also have psychological reactions, such as extreme *anxiety* (see Volume 2), delusions (false beliefs), or even feelings of persecution. In the most severe cases of amphetamine abuse users may behave in a psychotic manner, as if they were severely mentally ill.

Symptoms of Overuse. A person who is abusing amphetamines may be extremely irritable, have difficulty sleeping, and fail to eat. In some cases people on amphetamines can exhibit violent behaviors. The drugs can also cause HALLUCINATIONS or convulsions, and an overdose of amphetamines can be fatal.

AMYL NITRATE Also known as *poppers*, a drug sometimes used to treat ***high blood pressure*** (see Volume 8) and ASTHMA. Amyl nitrate is a fast-acting drug with effects felt within about 30 seconds of use. The drug lowers blood pressure and causes muscles to relax. At the same time, it also increases the heart rate. Amyl nitrate can cause severe headache as well as dizziness and nausea.

When abused, amyl nitrate is used to create a temporary high. It is thought to enhance sexual orgasms and is sometimes abused for this reason. The drug is very dangerous when abused or used without proper medical supervision because of its effect on lowering blood pressure and increasing heart rate. It can be especially dangerous for people who suffer from HEART DISEASE. The drug may also contribute to BRONCHITIS and cause sudden death in some users. [*See also* DRUGS AND HEALTH PROBLEMS.]

ANABOLIC STEROIDS Drugs that are synthetic versions of the male hormone testosterone. Anabolic steroids may be prescribed for males who have growth disorders or hormone deficiencies. However, they are sometimes used illegally by athletes or others, both male and female, who wish to increase muscle strength. Other types of *steroids* (see Volume 4) are used for stress, birth control, and hormone therapy.

Anabolic steroids can cause various side effects, including severe acne, *high blood pressure* (see Volume 8), and psychotic rages known as roid rage. Men using the drugs may experience early balding, impotence, shrunken testicles, and abnormal development of the breasts (a condition known as *gynecomastia*). Women who use anabolic steroids may experience increased growth of body hair growth, disruptions in their menstrual cycles, and decreased breast size. The drugs can impair fertility in both men and women. Anabolic steroids can also damage the heart as well as the liver. Adolescents who abuse anabolic steroids may disrupt normal bone growth. [*See also* DRUGS AND HEALTH PROBLEMS.]

ANGEL DUST See PCP.

ANGINA PECTORIS See Volume 8.

ANTABUSE A drug often used as treatment for ALCOHOLISM. Those who take Antabuse and consume even a small quantity of ALCOHOL will experience uncontrollable vomiting. The drug also causes severe headache and has been known to cause breathing problems and even coma or death. Antabuse can also cause HEPATITIS and liver disease in some people.

In recent years other medications, such as NALTREXONE, have been found to produce fewer complications than Antabuse and are also more effective in treating ALCOHOL ADDICTION. However, some experts believe that Antabuse, combined with other drugs, can still be effective in combating alcoholism. [*See also* ALCOHOLISM TREATMENT.]

ANTIBIOTICS DRUGS used to fight infections caused by bacteria, which are microscopic, one-celled organisms. Antibiotics work either by killing bacteria directly or by interfering with their reproductive cycle so they do not multiply. They are no help against infections caused by viruses, such as common colds, influenza, and most sore throats. Antibiotics can be very effective, however, against bacterial infections such as urinary tract infections, bacterial conjunctivitis, most ear infections, and infected cuts and scrapes. There are many different kinds of antibiotics, each one designed to target a particular type of bacteria or infectious disease.

Antibiotics do have some drawbacks. Like almost all drugs, they cause side effects (mostly mild ones like nausea, vomiting, and diarrhea). A greater risk is antibiotic resistance. If antibiotics are overused, or not used properly, the bacteria they are used against can become immune, or resistant, to the drug, rendering it ineffective. Then alternative antibiotics must be selected or developed. Despite such drawbacks, antibiotics continue to be used, and new ones are being created because experts recognize that antibiotics do work, and their overall impact on people's health has been positive. Antibiotics have saved hundreds of thousands of lives by destroying bacteria that cause infections and many serious diseases, including scarlet fever, diphtheria, and tuberculosis.

ANTISMOKING LAWS Laws designed to restrict smoking. Based on findings of the Surgeon General that TOBACCO causes cancer, federal and state governments have enacted various laws to restrict smoking. Many of these laws focus on protecting children and adolescents from tobacco products. For example, all states ban retailers from selling tobacco products to people under age 18, and in 23 states a retailer can lose his license if caught selling tobacco to a minor. The District of Columbia and 19 states ban cigarette vending machines in areas accessible to minors, and about half the states prohibit smoking in day-care centers.

Other antismoking laws are geared to protect all people, focusing primarily on providing cleaner air or restricting tobacco advertising. About 30 states have laws that restrict smoking in restaurants, and 41 states ban smoking inside government buildings. Federal laws ban smoking on most airline flights, and there are also laws that ban television ads that promote cigarettes.

ANTISMOKING PRODUCTS Products used by individuals in an attempt to stop smoking. Most antismoking products use NICOTINE REPLACEMENT THERAPY and come in the form of gum, nasal sprays, inhalers, and skin patches. Nicotine nasal sprays or nicotine inhalers are available by prescription only. Another effective antismoking product is the prescribed medication Zyban. The U.S. federal government is currently investigating the effectiveness of other alternative antismoking remedies as well.

Nicotine Replacement Products. It is easier for many people to stop smoking if they can still maintain some nicotine in their systems. A federal government analysis of studies on antismoking

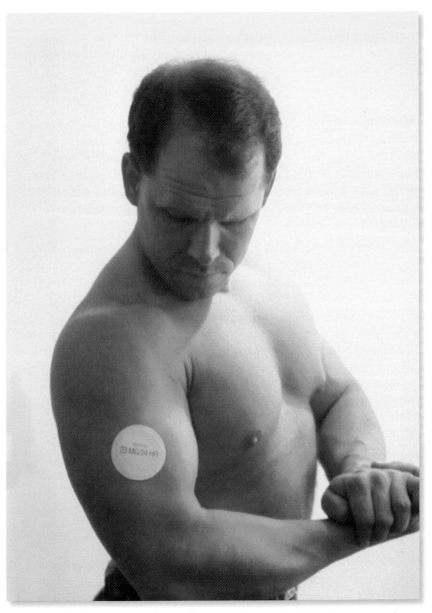

The skin patch, a form of nicotine replacement therapy, has helped many people stop smoking.

products found that many smokers had good success with nicotine gum, although nicotine patches, inhalers, or nasal sprays were all much more effective as antismoking agents.

People who use a nicotine replacement drug in any form should not continue to smoke. If they continue to smoke and also use the medications, the levels of nicotine in their bodies may rise to a dangerous level and could cause heart problems.

Nonnicotine Medications. Some prescribed medications that help smokers overcome their addiction to TOBACCO do not use nicotine. At present, Zyban Sustained Release (SR), also known as bupropion SR, is the only approved nonnicotine drug for SMOKING CESSATION. Some physicians prescribe other medications to help people stop smoking, although they are not specifically approved by the Food and Drug Administration (FDA) as nonsmoking remedies.

Alternative Remedies. The federal government is currently investigating whether herbal remedies or other forms of ALTERNATIVE MEDICINE may help people quit smoking. For example, studies on Chinese herbs, particularly the plant kudzu, may find that certain plants may be effective in helping smokers end their habit. Other treatments, such as acupuncture or HYPNOTHERAPY, may also be effective for the smoker who wants to quit. [*See also* ADDICTION, MEDICATIONS FOR.]

ASTHMA Chronic respiratory disease in which breathing becomes difficult because the airways of the lungs become narrowed or clogged as a result of swelling and a build-up of mucus. An asthma "attack" generally includes wheezing, a feeling of tightness in the chest, and shortness of breath. Most asthma attacks are provoked by allergies to pollen, pets, or other substances. Some experts believe that asthma may also be triggered by smoking and that smoking or exposure to smoke increases the severity of asthma attacks. [*See also* TOBACCO AND HEALTH PROBLEMS.]

BARBITURATES Medications derived from barbituric acid that have been prescribed by physicians since about 1900. Barbiturates act to slow down the central nervous system and are generally prescribed as sedatives or antiseizure medications. They may also be used to treat alcoholics who are going through the symptoms of WITHDRAWAL.

Regular or excessive use of barbiturates can lead to both abuse and addiction. When abused, barbiturates are particularly dangerous and can cause death when used in combination with ALCOHOL or taken in large doses. For those addicted to the drugs the withdrawal symptoms from barbiturates can be severe and can include nausea and vomiting, delirium, and convulsions.

BEER An alcoholic beverage brewed from grain and from hops, a flavoring agent. Beer is one of the most popular beverages in the United States. About 69 percent of all beer drinkers are men, and they drink about twice as much beer as women.

Most beers have an ALCOHOL content of 3–6 percent, although some have lower or higher alcohol contents. So-called lite beer is more popular among females. Lite beers have fewer calories than regular beer, but they do not have a lower alcohol content. In comparing different types of alcohol and their alcohol contents, 12 ounces of beer is equal to 1.5 ounces of 80-proof distilled spirits and to 5 ounces of wine.

Many people do not realize that abuse of beer can lead to ADDICTION as well as to major health problems such as cancer, CIRRHOSIS of the liver, HEART DISEASE, ALCOHOLIC BLACKOUTS, and HIGH BLOOD PRESSURE. Abuse of beer also lowers inhibitions and may thus lead people to unsafe sex, DRIVING WHILE INTOXICATED OR DRUG IMPAIRED, CHILD ABUSE, and criminal behavior. [*See also* ALCOHOL AND HEALTH PROBLEMS; CANCERS.]

BINGE DRINKING Drinking excessive amounts of ALCOHOL within a short period of time. Binge drinking is a form of ALCOHOL ABUSE that may lead to ALCOHOL ADDICTION. Experts define binge drinking as having five or more drinks on at least one day in the past 30 days.

According to a national survey on DRUG ABUSE, binge drinking reaches a peak at age 21 and then begins to decline. In 1999, 45 million Americans ages 12 and over engaged in binge drinking. Of these about 7 million were between ages 12 to 20.

Chugging is a form of binge drinking that involves consuming several drinks within seconds or minutes. Because the body is unable to metabolize, or process, the alcohol fast enough, chugging may lead to ALCOHOL POISONING and result in coma or death.

Although binge drinking can start in the early teen years, many binge drinkers are college students. A 1998 study of adolescents

Fact or Folklore?

Folklore Beer is not as bad for you as hard liquor.

Some people believe that as long as they drink only beer and no distilled spirits (such as whiskey or bourbon), then they do not have a risk for ALCOHOLISM or any health problems associated with alcohol. However, the facts are that heavy beer drinking is unhealthy and can be an indicator of alcoholism. Studies have also shown that heavy beer drinkers have a ten times greater risk of developing CANCER of the esophagus as do nondrinkers. Beer drinking can also contribute to or cause *obesity* (see Volume 4).

ages 12–17 revealed that nearly 8 percent were binge drinkers compared to about 17 percent of people over age 18.

Researchers have found racial differences for binge drinking. According to studies, about 11 percent of American Indian/Alaska Native adolescents ages 12–17 had engaged in binge drinking. Among Caucasians and African American adolescents in the same age group the figures were 7 percent and 3 percent, respectively.

There are also gender and age differences associated with binge drinking. Males have a greater problem with binge drinking than females. Among adolescents ages 12–17 about 9 percent of males are binge drinkers compared to about 7 percent of females. This gender gap widens greatly with age. About 25 percent of men over age 18 engage in binge drinking, compared to only about 9 percent of females in this age group.

There are also wide variations among states of levels of binge drinking. In 1999 North Dakota had the highest rate of binge drinking for people ages 12 and over (28.7 percent). Most states with high rates of binge drinking are in the northern parts of the United States, while most states with the lowest rates are in the South.

BLOOD ALCOHOL LEVELS A measurement of the percentage of alcohol in the blood; also known as **blood alcohol concentration (BAC)**. The BAC is used to determine legal INTOXICATION. Each state sets its own BAC limits, which range from 0.05 grams of alcohol per deciliter to 0.10 grams per deciliter.

According to a report by the Substance Abuse and Mental Health Services Administration (SAMHSA), in over 80 percent of car crashes resulting in fatalities the driver had a BAC that was more than 0.08 percent. A person who weighs about 170 pounds would have to drink over four drinks on an empty stomach in an hour to reach this level of intoxication. After California enacted 0.08 as their upper limit of blood alcohol levels, alcohol-related deaths dropped by 12 percent in the state.

There are special laws on blood alcohol levels for people who are under age 21. In response to an amendment to the National Minimum Drinking Age Act of 1995 all states and the District of Columbia passed ZERO TOLERANCE LAWS that established BAC limits for drivers under age 21 of either 0.00, 0.01, or 0.02.

BRONCHITIS An infection or irritation of the bronchial passages in the lungs that can be brought on or aggravated by smoking. The primary symptoms of bronchitis are severe coughing and an excessive production of mucus. People who smoke cigarettes are prone to frequent bouts of bronchitis. Moreover, the children

Keywords

blood alcohol concentration (BAC) the ratio of alcohol volume to blood volume in the body, expressed as a percent

malignant pertaining to cancerous cells that are likely to spread uncontrollably and to damage tissues of the body; cancerous

of people who smoke are more likely to have bronchitis than the children of nonsmokers. They are also more susceptible to colds and other respiratory ailments.

To treat bronchitis, physicians recommend the use of inhaler devices, as well as the use of humidifiers in the home. If the doctor believes the bronchitis stems from a *bacterial infection* (see Volume 8), he will generally prescribe an antibiotic. [*See also* TOBACCO AND HEALTH PROBLEMS.]

C

CANCERS Life-threatening **malignant** tumors. Certain *cancers* (see Volume 8) may stem from TOBACCO use, ALCOHOL ABUSE, excessive exposure to the *ultraviolet rays* (see Volume 6) of the sun, exposure to chemicals, or a combination of factors. People who both smoke and drink ALCOHOL increase the risk for cancer. The risks for contracting cancer also seem to have a genetic component, since certain cancers seem to run in families.

ADDICTION to tobacco contributes to many cases of LUNG CANCER and THROAT CANCER, two types of cancer closely associated with tobacco use. ALCOHOL ADDICTION can lead to cancer of the esophagus and rectal cancer, and women who are heavy drinkers are more prone to developing *breast cancer* (see Volume 8). Cancer is also linked to SECONDHAND SMOKE. According to the Surgeon General, exposure to secondhand smoke causes 3,000 lung cancer deaths per year among nonsmokers.

The primary symptoms of cancer can include the following: a thickening or lump in the breast or other part of the body, an obvious change in a mole or wart, a sore that does not heal, constant hoarseness or a nagging cough, a change in bowel or bladder habits, difficulty swallowing or indigestion, unexplained weight changes, and unusual discharges or bleeding. [*See also* ALCOHOL AND HEALTH PROBLEMS; TOBACCO AND HEALTH PROBLEMS.]

CANNABIS See HASHISH; MARIJUANA.

CARCINOGENS Substances known to cause CANCERS. Many of the ingredients found in TOBACCO are carcinogens. These substances may contribute to various forms of cancer, including ORAL CANCER, THROAT CANCER, and LUNG CANCER. Heavy and chronic use of alcohol may be linked to cancer as well. ALCOHOL ABUSE can cause alcohol to act as a carcinogen and can lead to cancers of the gastrointestinal system. [*See also* ALCOHOL AND HEALTH PROBLEMS; TOBACCO AND HEALTH PROBLEMS.]

CENTERS FOR DISEASE CONTROL AND PREVENTION (CDC) Federal agency in the U.S. Department of Health and Human Services that is responsible for investigating and helping to control diseases and disabilities. The CDC gathers data on the incidence of disease, helps determine the cause of epidemics and other health problems, and promotes ways to protect public health and prevent disease and disability. It also provides the latest information on diseases and public health to consumers, scientists, and government officials. The CDC maintains a dozen centers and offices that are concerned with different aspects of public health. The mission of the Division of Adolescent and School Health, a branch of the National Center for Chronic Disese Prevention and Health Promotion (NCCDHP), is to prevent serious health risk behaviors—such as drinking, smoking, and using ILLEGAL DRUGS—among adolescents. The Office of Smoking and Health (OSH), another division of the NCCDHP, concentrates on leading efforts to prevent tobacco use and promote SMOKING CESSATION. In addition, the National Center for Health Statistics compiles, analyzes, and provides statistical data on the abuse of tobacco, alcohol, and drugs, as well as other health topics.

MORE SOURCES See www.cdc.gov

CHEWING TOBACCO See SMOKELESS TOBACCO.

CHILD ABUSE Physical or sexual harm to children that is severe enough that it may warrant the child's temporary or permanent removal from the family. Child neglect is a form of *child abuse* (see Volume 5). A child is neglected when a parent does not provide for the child's basic needs, such as food and shelter. Each year thousands of children are removed from their homes because of abuse and neglect and placed in the foster care system.

ALCOHOL ABUSE and DRUG ABUSE are contributing factors in at least half of all cases of child abuse and neglect in the United States. Experts estimate that as many as two-thirds of all incidents of child abuse can be attributed to the abuse of either ALCOHOL or

<table>
<tr><td>**Keywords**</td></tr>
<tr><td>**anesthetic** drug that produces anesthesia, an insensitivity to pain and other sensations
child neglect failure to provide food, shelter, and medical attention; abandonment is a form of child neglect</td></tr>
</table>

DRUGS. Parents who are intoxicated or drugged may not intend or even realize that they are being abusive or neglectful. Nevertheless, children are sometimes severely abused and even murdered by parents and other caregivers who are under the influence of alcohol or other drugs.

The sexual abuse of children is also linked to the abuse of alcohol and drugs. An estimated one-third of all *sexual assaults* (see Volume 5) on children occurred when the adult committing the abuse was under the influence of alcohol. Adults who abuse alcohol or drugs are also more likely to commit crimes of DOMESTIC VIOLENCE AND ABUSE, especially of a spouse or lover.

CIGARETTES See TOBACCO.

CIGARS See TOBACCO.

CIRRHOSIS Serious *liver disease* (see Volume 8) characterized by severe and chronic inflammation of and damage to the liver. Cirrhosis of the liver is often due to chronic, long-term ALCOHOL ABUSE or ALCOHOL ADDICTION. Symptoms of the early stages of the disease are often difficult to identify. Only in the late stages are physical symptoms apparent. These symptoms include jaundice (a yellowish appearance of the skin), painful abdominal swelling, and confused behavior.

Cirrhosis of the liver can be diagnosed through a physical examination and laboratory tests of the blood. People with the disease are urged to stop consuming ALCOHOL completely. Although ABSTINENCE will not cure cirrhosis, it may slow the deterioration and damage to the liver. [*See also* ALCOHOL AND HEALTH PROBLEMS.]

CLUB DRUGS Popular and usually ILLEGAL DRUGS that are often consumed at all-night dance parties, some of which are called RAVES. The term *club drugs* is sometimes used interchangeably with DESIGNER DRUGS, which are synthetically produced drugs such as ECSTASY.

According to the National Institute on Drug Abuse, popular club drugs include ALCOHOL, LSD, Ecstasy (MDMA), AMPHETAMINES, and METHAMPHETAMINES. Club drugs may also include what are generally referred to as DATE RAPE DRUGS, such as Rohypnol and GHB.

With the exception of alcohol, all club drugs are illegal drugs. Some of them, such as Ecstasy and various date rape drugs, are considered *designer drugs* because they were synthetically derived (or "designed") from another drug.

Club drugs can be extremely dangerous, especially when combined with other drugs or with alcohol. Many people have become extremely ill, permanently disabled, or have even died from consuming club drugs or from mixing them with alcohol or other drugs. [*See also* ALCOHOL AND HEALTH PROBLEMS.]

COCAINE Drug made from the leaves of the coca plant, which is native to South America; also called *blow* or *snow*. Cocaine is a STIMULANT that is highly addictive. It is also considered a NARCOTIC by the DRUG ENFORCEMENT ADMINISTRATION (DEA).

Cocaine is known primarily for its illegal use by people seeking to attain a "high," or feeling of euphoria. This feeling of intense elation is brief, usually lasting from 5 to 20 minutes. People ingest the drug by either sniffing it (also known as snorting) or by injecting it (a method known as MAINLINING). One popular form of cocaine known as CRACK COCAINE is smoked.

Cocaine has been used for hundreds of years. As early as the 1500s, and probably much earlier, priests among the Inca peoples of Peru sought religious experiences by chewing coca leaves, the source of cocaine. Throughout the following centuries people experimented with the drug and learned how to make a powdered form that could be sniffed.

At one time cocaine use was restricted to a relatively small group of adults. By 1998 an estimated 1.7 million Americans reported using cocaine at least once a month, with the largest percent of users between ages 18 and 25. In recent years cocaine use has been on the rise among youth. The percentage of high school seniors in the United States who used cocaine at least once has increased from 5.9 percent in 1994 to 9.8 percent in 1999. Usage among younger students has also increased. Among eighth graders cocaine use rose from 2.3 percent in 1991 to 4.7 percent in 1999.

Effects of Cocaine. Cocaine acts as both an **anesthetic**, depressing feelings in the nerve endings, and a STIMULANT, stimulating the central nervous system. The drug increases the heart rate and raises blood pressure and body temperature. Although users may feel highly energetic and elated after using cocaine, they feel extremely exhausted and depressed when the effect of the drug wears off. Users may also lose interest in sex or food.

Health Problems Caused by Cocaine. First-time users of cocaine risk experiencing fatal heart attacks because of the added strain the drug puts on the heart by causing heart rate to increase. People who sniff cocaine regularly may lose their sense of smell and suffer from frequent nosebleeds. Runny noses are common among cocaine abusers.

HEALTH UPDATE

Combining Alcohol and Cocaine
The combination of COCAINE and ALCOHOL is particularly dangerous and can lead to death. These two substances interact with each other to produce a chemical called cocaethylene. This chemical lasts longer and is more toxic than either cocaine or alcohol alone.

Other health consequences of cocaine besides an increased risk for heart attack include heart rhythm disturbances, or *arrhythmia* (see Volume 8), chest pain, respiratory failure, *stroke* (see Volume 8), headaches, abdominal pain, nausea, and seizures. Cocaine users who inject themselves intravenously risk contracting HIV or HEPATITIS. WITHDRAWAL from cocaine can cause *depression* (see Volume 2) and exhaustion.

Cocaine can also have harmful psychological effects on users. These include mood disturbances, paranoia, and auditory HALLUCINATIONS—hearing voices that are not really there. One uniquely dreadful complication of cocaine use is coke bugs, or parasitosis. This is a hallucination that many insects are crawling over or under the skin. Chronic cocaine users may also lapse into cocaine psychosis, in which they lose all touch with normal activities and with reality itself. [*See also* DRUGS AND HEALTH PROBLEMS.]

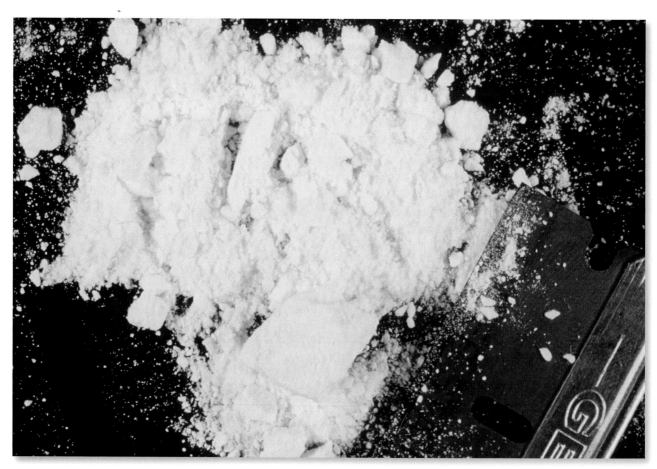

The powdered form of cocaine is ingested by sniffing or "snorting."

CODEPENDENCY A usually unspoken agreement or relationship between an addict and nonaddicted family members that unwittingly supports the addict's behavior or pretends that the ADDICTION does not exist. In codependent relationships any problems that are caused by the addiction are generally covered up by family members. An addict may also blame family members for his or her addictive behavior.

Nonaddicted family members in a codependent relationship may take over roles that the addict formerly held, such as primary wage earner. They may also handle responsibilities once undertaken regularly by the addict, such as cooking, child care, yard work, and other tasks. Family members in codependent relationships may receive physical or emotional abuse from the addicted person but not react to it because they feel both hopeless and helpless in the face of the addiction.

Children in families affected by codependency may blame themselves for the behavior of addicted parents. They may think that if they were only better behaved, more intelligent, or had some other attribute, then the addictive behavior would stop. These children may also harbor feelings of intense anger or *anxiety* (see Volume 2).

Organizations such as ALCOHOLICS ANONYMOUS (AA), AL-ANON, and ALATEEN help families break out of codependent patterns of behavior so that addicts will be forced to face the consequences of their actions. In fact, an important part of treating addictive behavior is for family members not to accept the addict's behavior. For example, if an alcoholic does not go to work because of a hangover, other family members should not call the workplace to explain or make excuses. That should be the responsibility of the addict.

CRACK COCAINE A form of cocaine that can be smoked, rather than injected or snorted, after FREEBASING, a process in which the cocaine is converted into a smokeable form. The substance is called "crack" because it makes a crackling sound when smoked.

First introduced in the mid-1980s in New York City, crack cocaine spread rapidly to other parts of the United States. In 1998 an estimated 437,000 Americans used crack. While most users are inner-city drug addicts, some reports indicate that urban teenagers also smoke crack along with MARIJUANA.

Crack cocaine is sold in chunks or rock forms, ready to be freebased. The drug is usually smoked using a water pipe, a device that helps to make the smoke less harsh to the throat. Crack is highly addictive and can lead to ADDICTION on the first use. The effects of the drug are similar to those caused by co-caine that is injected: dilated pupils of the eyes, increased body temperature and blood pressure, and hyperactivity. The user experiences a "high," or feeling of euphoria, in under ten seconds, which is one of the reasons for the drug's popularity among drug abusers.

Frequent use of crack cocaine can cause HALLUCINATIONS, insomnia, and a very intense form of paranoia. Crack use can also cause seizures or *cardiac arrest* (see Volume 8), which may result in death. The use of crack cocaine by a pregnant woman may be harmful to a developing fetus. Children born addicted to crack may have learning disabilities and attention deficit disorders, which affect their ability to concentrate on anything for long periods. [*See also* DRUGS AND HEALTH PROBLEMS.]

D

DATE RAPE DRUGS Drugs that can be placed into the drink of an unknowing person in order to cause disorientation and to make the victim susceptible to *sexual assault and rape* (see Volume 3). The term *date rape drugs* is commonly used to refer to drugs such as Rohypnol, GHB (gamma hydroxybutyrate), Klonopin (clonazepam), and ketamine. These drugs are colorless, tasteless, and odorless and are therefore impossible for the victim to detect. Special urine tests can detect the presence of these drugs in the body, but only if testing is done within 72 hours after a drug has been ingested.

Victims and Effects of the Drugs. Date rape victims can be either male or female, and the drugs have been administered illegally to others by both heterosexuals and homosexuals. Date rape drugs typically have a rapid sedative effect on the central nervous system, acting within about 15 minutes to make the victim drowsy and disoriented. The drugs also have amnesiac qualities, which means that the victim will have difficulty remembering (or cannot remember at all) what occurred while under the influence of the drug.

Shortly after unknowingly taking a date rape drug, the victim appears intoxicated to others. The appearance of INTOXICATION allows the assailant to convince any others present that the victim needs to leave. While the victim is drowsy and disoriented, the assailant has the opportunity to commit assault or rape. When assaulted persons later return to normal, they may become suspicious, perhaps because they find themselves in a strange place with their clothes off or rumpled. However, since they can remember little or nothing of what happened, they are uncertain how to act.

In 1996 Congress passed the Drug-Induced Rape Prevention and Punishment Act. This law increased the punishments associated with controlled drugs to as many as 20 years when they are used without another person's knowledge in order to commit an act of sexual assault, rape, or violence against that person.

Common Date Rape Drugs. One of the most common date rape drugs is Rohypnol (flunitrazepam). Illegal in the United States, this drug is sold legally in other countries as a remedy for insomnia or as a preanesthetic drug. Its effects include dizziness, drowsiness, lack of coordination, and gastrointestinal disturbances that last for at least 12 hours after taking the drug.

Another drug associated with sexual assaults is gamma hydroxybutyrate (GHB). Originally sold legally, this drug, illegal since 1992, was often abused by bodybuilders as well as individuals seeking its sedative or euphoric effects. Also known as liquid ecstasy, the drug can cause seizures, respiratory arrest (an end to breathing), and sometimes death.

Another date rape drug is ketamine, an anesthetic most commonly used by veterinarians. The drug has a rapid sedating effect and can cause HALLUCINATIONS similar to those produced by PCP. [*See also* CLUB DRUGS; DESIGNER DRUGS.]

DEATH FROM ADDICTIONS Fatalities caused by ADDICTION to ALCOHOL, TOBACCO, and other DRUGS. Addiction to or abuse of drugs, alcohol, or tobacco causes thousands of deaths each year in the United States. Many people do not realize the cost of these addictions in terms of lives lost and shortened. Few smokers know, for example, that they lose approximately seven minutes of life for every cigarette smoked. For most smokers this amounts to about 7 to 13 years of their lives that are smoked away. An addiction to drugs also take lives. About one-third of all deaths from *AIDS* (see Volume 7) are directly related to drug use, often from sharing needles with injection-drug users.

> ## VICTIMS OF COMBINING DRUGS WITH ALCOHOL
>
> People who abuse alcohol are more likely to use illegal drugs. Combining alcohol with other drugs resulted in the deaths of 3,723 people in the United States in 1998.

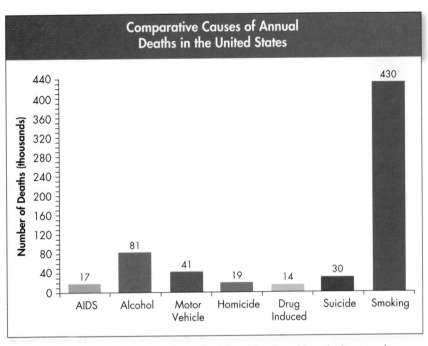

Comparative Causes of Annual Deaths in the United States

[Source: Centers for Disease Control and Prevention, *Tobacco Information and Prevention Source*, 1999.]

Alcohol-related Deaths. Experts estimate that ALCOHOL ADDICTION or ALCOHOL ABUSE is a factor in at least half of all adult *drownings* (see Volume 5) and fatal falls. Male alcoholics have a risk of injury-related death that is two to eight times greater than nonalcoholic men. They also have a five-times greater risk of dying from *motor vehicle injuries* (see Volume 5) sustained in a car crash. In addition, alcoholics are at greater risk for developing life-threatening diseases such as CANCER, *coronary heart disease* (see Volume 8), and *stroke* (see Volume 8).

Drug-related Deaths. Thousands of people die each year as a result of abusing drugs. Males are three times more likely to die from drug use than females. Death rates also differ by ethnic and racial background. About 61 percent of drug-related deaths occur among whites, with African Americans and Hispanics making up 27 percent and 10 percent respectively.

According to data reported in the year 2000 for major cities across the nation, COCAINE caused or contributed to the most drug-related deaths in the United States in 1998. The next most significant drug in terms of drug-related deaths was HEROIN. Among unintentional (nonsuicidal) deaths cocaine and heroin were again the leading substances involved, followed by alcohol in combination with a drug. Meanwhile, in drug-related *suicides* (see Volumes 2, 5) the substances most commonly associated with taking one's own life were alcohol in combination with another drug (34 percent) and cocaine (25 percent).

Many people who abuse drugs use more than one substance, and about 65 percent of drug-related deaths are caused by overdoses of multiple drugs. Among youths ages 12–17, 62 percent of drug-related deaths were not caused solely by drugs but involved a combination of drug use and an external physical event, usually a car crash. Some drug-related deaths are caused by legally prescribed drugs. The drugs most commonly associated with such deaths are codeine, Valium, and METHADONE.

Death and Tobacco. TOBACCO ADDICTION costs 430,000 lives in the United States each year. Yet tobacco-related deaths are the single most preventable cause of death in the nation. Of the approximately 160,000 deaths annually from LUNG CANCER, at least 90 percent can be attributed directly to tobacco. Moreover, the federal government estimates that about half of all deaths of male smokers—from any cause—can be attributed to cigarette smoking. Most of these men die of heart attack, cancer, or stroke—all of which are linked to smoking. Among female smokers 43 percent of all deaths are associated with smoking.

Alcoholism and Smoking Deaths. The overwhelming majority of people with ALCOHOLISM are also heavy smokers. Thus many alcoholics die from smoking-related diseases such as lung cancer, THROAT CANCER, EMPHYSEMA, and heart attacks. Some studies have found that more alcoholics die from smoking-related diseases than alcoholism-related illnesses. [*See also* HEART DISEASE.]

DELIRIUM TREMENS (DTs)

A serious condition suffered by some people with long-term ALCOHOL ADDICTION as they go through the physical WITHDRAWAL from ALCOHOL. Also known as "DTs" or "complicated alcohol abstinence," delirium tremens can also be triggered by heavy ALCOHOL ABUSE combined with inadequate food intake.

The common symptoms of delirium tremens are confusion; HALLUCINATIONS (often of bugs or snakes); heavy sweating; seizures; nausea and vomiting; fever; pale skin; *anxiety* (see Volume 2); insomnia; extreme sensitivity to sound, light, and touch; and extremely changeable emotions. Symptoms may last for several days or for weeks. In a small number of cases patients remain in a state of PSYCHOSIS after other symptoms subside.

People with delirium tremens require hospitalization because a severe case of the DTs can lead to heart attack and even death. Physicians generally treat individuals suffering from delirium tremens with sedatives or antianxiety medications. They may also administer antipsychotic medications to treat severe hallucinations.

While in the hospital, individuals suffering from delirium tremens will be tested for *liver disease* (see Volume 8) and vitamin deficiencies, which are very common among severely ill alcoholics. Doctors will also urge those treated for the DTs to practice complete ABSTINENCE from alcohol, and they often encourage them to seek help from organizations such as ALCOHOLICS ANONYMOUS (AA). [*See also* ALCOHOL AND HEALTH PROBLEMS.]

DEPENDENCE, PHYSICAL Recognizable physical symptoms of ADDICTION. The symptoms of physical dependence vary with the substance. For example, frequent MARIJUANA users often have reddened eyes, while COCAINE abusers often have a chronic runny nose or other nasal problems. Some symptoms become more apparent when the user is deprived of a substance and experiences WITHDRAWAL. Typical withdrawal symptoms range from sweating and headache to more serious DELIRIUM TREMENS (DTs) and seizures. In the most severe cases withdrawal from a substance can result in coma or death.

The degree of physical dependence varies according to the substance and the degree of addiction. For example, CRACK COCAINE or HEROIN can cause a very strong physical dependence, as can ALCOHOL. As a result, the withdrawal symptoms associated with these substances can be so severe that hospitalization is required and the individual must undergo DETOXIFICATION. Individuals with a physical dependence on tobacco will also experience withdrawal symptoms such as severe headache and agitation. Most people can undergo detoxification from TOBACCO with the help of a physician. [*See also* DEPENDENCE, PSYCHOLOGICAL; TOLERANCE, PHYSICAL.]

DEPENDENCE, PSYCHOLOGICAL An intense emotional need or craving for ALCOHOL, TOBACCO, or DRUGS. Psychological dependence is a stage of ADDICTION that may proceed to more advanced stages, including tolerance and physical dependence. Individuals who are dependent on alcohol, tobacco, or drugs may experience psychological distress and become agitated and anxious when deprived of the substance. But those who are psychologically dependent on these substances do not necessarily have a physical dependence on them, nor will they experience the physical symptoms associated with WITHDRAWAL if they stop taking the substances. [*See also* DEPENDENCE, PHYSICAL; TOLERANCE, PHYSICAL.]

DEPRESSANTS Drugs that depress or slow down the central nervous system. Depressant drugs include ALCOHOL, OPIATES, tranquilizers, and BARBITURATES. When used legally as medications, depressants are often taken to relieve tension and *anxiety* (see Volume 2). Many people use alcohol to achieve these same results. Depressants may also have a temporary mood-elevating effect because they slow down the nervous system.

Abuse of nonalcohol depressants can cause behaviors that resemble alcoholic INTOXICATION, such as staggering and slurred speech as well as poor judgment. The person may also have dilated (enlarged) pupils of the eyes. Among the signs of an overdose of depressant drugs are clammy skin, weak or very rapid pulse, and shallow breathing.

When people who are addicted to nonalcohol depressants stop taking them, they will experience symptoms of WITHDRAWAL such as extreme anxiety, insomnia, and a lack of appetite. Quickly stopping consumption of the drug, or dropping rapidly from a high dosage to a lower one, can cause convulsions and death.

Among the consequences of ALCOHOL ABUSE are ALCOHOL ADDICTION and a broad array of health problems, such as CIRRHOSIS

Commonly Abused Drugs: Depressants

Substances	Examples of Proprietary or Street Names	Medical Uses	Route of Administration	DEA Schedules*	Period of Detection
ALCOHOL	BEER, WINE, LIQUOR	ANTIDOTE FOR METHANOL POISONING	ORAL	NOT SCHEDULED	6–10 HOURS
BARBITURATES	AMYTAL, NEMBUTAL, SECONAL, PHENOBARBITAL; BARBS	ANTICONVULSANT, HYPNOTIC, SEDATIVE	INJECTED, ORAL	II, III, IV	2–10 DAYS
BENZODIAZEPINES	ATIVAN, HALCION, LIBRIUM, ROHYPNOL, VALIUM; ROOFIES, TRANKS, XANAX	ANTIANXIETY, ANTICONVULSANT, HYPNOTIC, SEDATIVE	INJECTED, ORAL	IV	1–6 WEEKS
METHAQUALONE	QUAALUDE	NONE	ORAL	I	2 WEEKS

*Drug Enforcement Administration (DEA) Schedule I and II drugs have a high potential for abuse. They require greater storage security and have a quota on manufacture, among other restrictions. Schedule I drugs are available for research only and have no approved medical use. Schedule II drugs are available only through prescription, cannot have refills, and require a form for ordering. Schedule III and IV drugs are available with prescription, may have five refills in six months, and may be ordered verbally. Most Schedule V drugs are available over the counter.

[Source: National Institute on Drug Abuse, *Sixth Annual Report to Congress*, 2001.]

of the liver, HIGH BLOOD PRESSURE, and HEART DISEASE. [*See also* ALCOHOL AND HEALTH PROBLEMS; DRUGS AND HEALTH PROBLEMS.]

DESIGNER DRUGS Synthetic ILLEGAL DRUGS that are derived from existing drugs such as METHAMPHETAMINES, MESCALINE, and the pain-relievers meperidine and fentanyl. Designer drugs are often referred to as CLUB DRUGS because adolescents and young adults frequently use them at private night clubs or at RAVES. In the 1990s designer drugs became increasingly popular in the United States, particularly in the West and the Southwest. Although the drugs are very popular, few users are aware of the serious health risks associated with them.

Perhaps the most well-known designer drug is MDMA (methylenedioxymethampetamine), more commonly known as ECSTASY. A PSYCHOACTIVE DRUG that produces effects similar to STIMULANTS and HALLUCINOGENS, this drug is derived from methamphetamines. Use of Ecstasy can cause nausea, HALLUCINATIONS, chills, sweating, tremors, increases in body temperature, muscle cramping, and blurred vision. Long-term use of the drug can lead to *depression, anxiety* (see Volume 2), paranoia, memory loss, and permanent brain damage.

Herbal Ecstasy, a variation of Ecstasy, is a designer drug derived from the stimulant ephedrine (*ma huang*) or from pseudoephedrine and caffeine. This very dangerous drug, sold in tablet form, can cause heart attacks, seizures, brain damage, and death. Because Herbal Ecstasy is considered a "natural" herbal substance, users may mistakenly assume that the drug is safe. They may also take extra doses or combine it with ALCOHOL and other drugs.

PMA (paramethoxyamphetamine) is another very dangerous designer drug, one that is much more toxic than Ecstasy. PMA is also known on the street as "Death," and a number of deaths among adolescents and young adults have been attributed to the drug. Doses of more than 50 milligrams of PMA can cause irregular heartbeats, heart attacks, breathing difficulties, kidney failure, convulsions, coma, and death. Death generally occurs when PMA is combined with other drugs and when body temperature rises so high that it causes the central nervous system to shut down.

DETOXIFICATION The process of ridding the body of an addicting substance, usually done in a hospital or a residential facility for drug addicts or alcoholics. Experts emphasize that detoxification is only a first step to treatment for ADDICTION. Most substance abusers also need intensive counseling as well as help from such organizations as ALCOHOLICS ANONYMOUS (AA) or Narcotics Anonymous.

Detoxification is a difficult process because the addict must undergo WITHDRAWAL and experience the symptoms associated with it. Depending on the addicting substance, these symptoms may range from fever, shakiness, and agitation to more severe symptoms such as HALLUCINATIONS and seizures. To lessen some of the withdrawal symptoms brought on by detoxification, physicians may prescribe various medications, often tranquilizers such as Valium or Librium. [*See also* ALCOHOL AND DRUG REHABILITATION PROGRAMS.]

DOMESTIC VIOLENCE AND ABUSE Physical harm to a spouse, intimate partner, child, or other family member or individual living in the home. Violence against a family member is much more likely to occur when the perpetrator of the abuse is under the influence of ALCOHOL or DRUGS. Incidents of CHILD ABUSE are also found much more frequently in families in which ALCOHOL ABUSE and DRUG ABUSE are common.

The use of drugs or alcohol apparently decreases the ability of adults to cope with the everyday needs of family members and the demands of domestic life. Use of the substances raises the irritability levels of abusers, for whom even simple requests may seem intolerable. The abusers respond by lashing out at those around them.

According to statistics compiled by the Bureau of Justice Statistics, alcohol and drugs play a very large role in domestic violence. In 1998, for example, in 57 percent of physical assaults against a current or former domestic partner the attacker had consumed alcohol beforehand. In 11 percent of the cases the abuser had consumed both alcohol and drugs, while in 8 percent of the cases the attacker had consumed only drugs.

Studies have also shown that physical aggression between newly married couples is four times more likely to involve alcohol (with the husband drinking) than when verbal arguments occur. Distressed couples who do not drink are more likely to vent their anger verbally. If alcohol is involved in domestic disputes, violence becomes a much greater risk. Studies have shown that domestic violence decreases significantly after an individual receives treatment for ALCOHOLISM, and the improvement sticks if the alcoholic continues to practice ABSTINENCE from alcohol.

DRINKING AND DRIVING See DRIVING WHILE INTOXICATED OR DRUG IMPAIRED.

DRINKING IN COLLEGE Abuse of ALCOHOL on college campuses. College students between the ages of 18 and 22 are heavier drinkers than nonstudent adults of the same age. About 63 percent of full-time college students use alcohol, compared to 52

Binge Drinking among College Students

Characteristics	Percent binge drinkers			Percent frequent binge drinkers*		
	1993	1997	1999	1993	1997	1999
ALL STUDENTS	44.5%	42.9%	44.1%	19.8%	20.9%	22.7%
SEX						
MALES	50.7	48.5	50.7	22.8	23.8	26.0
FEMALES	39.9	39.3	40.0	17.5	19.0	20.6
RACE ETHNICITY						
WHITE	48.4	45.9	49.2	22.0	23.5	26.3
BLACK	15.7	19.1	15.5	6.4	6.6	6.5
ASIAN/PACIFIC ISLANDER	22.1	25.3	23.1	7.6	9.4	8.4
OTHER	38.8	37.4	39.6	15.4	17.2	17.4
HISPANIC	39.0	37.9	39.5	15.4	17.2	16.6
NON-HISPANIC	44.8	43.3	44.5	20.1	21.3	23.2
AGE						
23 YEARS OR YOUNGER	47.5	45.6	47.0	22.0	21.3	24.8
24 YEARS OR OLDER	29.0	28.8	28.1	8.8	9.7	10.8
YEARS IN SCHOOL						
FRESHMAN	49.5	43.3	42.1	21.1	23.1	22.3
SOPHOMORE	45.7	43.8	44.5	20.1	22.5	24.1
JUNIOR	44.7	44.5	45.9	20.2	20.9	23.2
SENIOR	44.0	41.3	44.9	19.4	18.7	22.3
RESIDENCE						
DORMITORY	47.3	45.3	44.5	22.5	22.5	23.0
FRATERNITY/SORORITY HOUSE	83.1	81.6	78.9	49.4	52.5	51.1
OFF CAMPUS	41.1	40.2	43.7	17.0	18.8	22.1
FRATERNITY/SORORITY MEMBER	87.4	65.5	64.7	34.3	38.6	39.6
BINGED IN HIGH SCHOOL						
NO	32.3	30.9	31.1	10.9	11.3	12.2
YES	69.7	70.7	73.9	38.2	43.3	46.7
MARITAL STATUS						
NEVER MARRIED	47.5	45.7	45.9	21.7	22.8	24.4
MARRIED	20.5	18.7	18.3	4.7	5.3	6.4

*Students who binged three or more times in the previous 2-week period.

[Source: Henry Wechesler et al., *Journal of American College Health*, 2000.]

percent of young adults not in college. One of the major alcohol-related problems on college campuses is BINGE DRINKING.

Heavy and Binge Drinking. Collegiate males are heavier drinkers than females. In a 1999 survey of national drug use, about 17 percent of male college students reported heavy drinking compared to about 11 percent of female students. Males also had more episodes of binge drinking. Of those who reported heavy drinking, about 53 percent of the men had engaged in binges compared to 34 percent of the women.

In 1999 the Harvard School of Public Health studied college students and drinking at 199 colleges in 39 states. The majority of those who responded to the study were female (61 percent). The researchers found that 44 percent of the students were binge drinkers, about 39 percent were non-binge drinkers, and 19 percent did not drink alcohol at all. The binge drinkers were about evenly divided between occasional binge drinkers (22 percent) and frequent binge drinkers (21 percent).

The Harvard researchers further analyzed the college binge drinkers and found that for a majority of these students (74 percent), their drinking problems began before they entered college. There was also a distinctive difference among where the binge drinkers lived compared to others. Seventy-nine percent of those who lived in a fraternity or sorority house were binge drinkers, a figure that contrasted sharply with the 44.5 percent of binge drinkers living in a dormitory and 44 who lived off campus.

Risky Behavior. According to the Harvard study, the heavy drinking and bingeing students had much higher rates of risky behavior. Only about 4 percent of the nonbinge drinkers engaged in *unprotected sex* (see Volume 3) compared to 10 percent for occasional binge drinkers and 20 percent of frequent binge drinkers. The study clearly showed a strong link between drinking and unsafe sex.

Nearly 57 percent of the frequent binge drinkers also admitted to driving a car after drinking alcohol. In comparison, about 40 percent of the occasional binge drinkers drove while intoxicated, and only about 19 percent of the nonbinge drinkers did. The least safe drivers were thus most likely to drive drunk.

The Harvard Study and other studies on college students and heavy or binge drinking clearly show that drinking alcohol contributes to very high risk behaviors among some college students. These behaviors not only endanger themselves but others as well. [*See also* ALCOHOL OVERDOSE; ALCOHOL POISONING; DRIVING WHILE INTOXICATED OR DRUG IMPAIRED.]

DRIVING WHILE INTOXICATED OR DRUG IMPAIRED

Driving a motor vehicle while under the influence of ALCOHOL or DRUGS, also known as *driving under the influence (dui)*. **Drunk driving** (see Volume 5) is a serious problem in the United States. In 1998, for example, alcohol was a factor in 38 percent of all car crash fatalities. In 40 percent of these deaths the person who died was not intoxicated but was a passenger or a pedestrian hit by an alcohol-impaired driver.

Younger Drivers. Younger drivers are at greatest risk for dying from driving while intoxicated. Drivers under age 21 are twice as likely to be killed as a result of drunk driving than older drivers. Younger drivers are also more likely to drive while drug-impaired. In one study nearly a million youths from ages 16 to 18 reported driving a vehicle within two hours of using an illegal drug. Compounding the problem of driving while intoxicated or drug-impaired is the fact that younger drivers have less driving experience and thus are less able to handle a car well in a problem situation.

Decreases in Risk. In general there has been a decrease in drunk driving over the last few decades, as indicated by statistics on driving and BLOOD ALCOHOL LEVELS (also known as **blood alcohol concentrations (BACs)**. In 1973, for example, 10.9 percent of the drivers ages 15–20 stopped for drunk driving had BACs of 0.05 and 4.1 percent had BACs of 0.10. The public became alarmed at

Percent of Drivers with High BACs

	BAC 0.05			BAC 0.10		
AGE	1973	1985	1996	1973	1985	1996
15–20	10.9	4.6	2.8	4.1	2.7	0.3
21–34	15.4	9.9	11.3	5.7	3.3	3.8
35–44	15.9	9.4	6.9	5.8	4.7	3.7
45+	12.1	6.8	5.2	4.1	1.8	1.7
Sex						
MALES	14.7	9.9	8.7	5.5	3.9	3.5
FEMALES	8.8	3.9	5.8	3.0	1.3	1.5
Ethnic						
HISPANIC	22.0	13.0	14.9	3.3	4.4	7.5
WHITE	13.3	7.4	7.1	5.1	2.7	2.3
BLACK	16.5	13.5	9.4	6.0	5.9	3.6

[U.S. Department of Transportation, National Highway Safety Administration, 2000.]

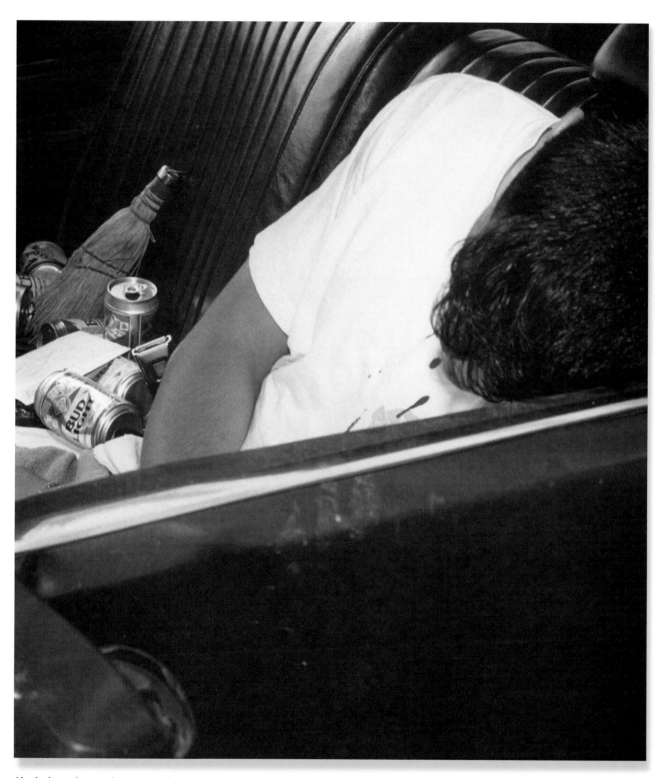

Alcohol use is a major cause of car crash fatalities in the United States.

these high rates, and groups such as *MADD (Mothers Against Drunk Driving)* (see Volume 5) argued for strong actions against drunk driving. By 1986 the situation had improved considerably, and the numbers for the same blood alcohol levels dropped to 4.6 and 2.7 percent respectively. Law officials have also enacted a greater amount of sobriety checkpoints in order to catch people who drive while intoxicated or drug-impaired.

Driving while intoxicated has continued to decrease among younger drivers. By 1996, for example, only 2.8 percent of these drivers had a BAC of 0.05 and only 0.3 percent had a BAC of 0.10. However, the situation has worsened for some groups over the same time period. For example, since 1986 there has been an increase in the percentage of drunken driving among females and Hispanics ages 21–34.

Zero Tolerance Laws. In an effort to further reduce car crashes among young people, many states have passed so-called ZERO TOLERANCE LAWS. Since 1998 all states have had such laws, which label legal INTOXICATION as blood alcohol levels of between zero and 0.02. By lowering the acceptable levels even more, these laws may prove to be a major deterrent against drunk driving.

VICTIMS OF DRUG ABUSE

Researchers have found varying patterns among drug abusers based on such factors as age, race, sex, education, and geographic location, as well as on the particular substance abused. For example, IN-HALANTS are abused primarily by adolescents. Among white adolescents ages 12–17 an estimated 3.4 percent have abused inhalants, compared to only 1 percent of whites in other age groups. Among Hispanics and African Americans of the same age the figures are 2.8 percent and about 1 percent respectively.

Drug use also seems to vary geographically. Some states, for example, have higher rates of DRUG ABUSE than others. In 1999 Alaska reported the highest rate of substance abuse, with 7.3 percent of the population over age 12 dependent on drugs or alcohol and 2.8 percent dependent on ILLEGAL DRUGS.

DRUG ABUSE Excessive use of legal or ILLEGAL DRUGS. Despite efforts to curtail drug use, drug abuse remains a serious problem in the United States. For some users drug abuse may lead to DRUG ADDICTION. This can often occur very quickly. With CRACK CO-CAINE, for example, ADDICTION can occur after only the first use of the substance. With some other drugs, however, it may take months or years for an addition to develop. In general, males abuse drugs at about twice the rate of females.

Drugs of Abuse. The drugs most abused in the U.S. today are MARIJUANA, COCAINE, HEROIN, METHAMPHETAMINE, and CLUB DRUGS such as ECSTASY. Many people combine drugs with ALCOHOL, which can be particularly dangerous. For example, the combination of cocaine and alcohol can be fatal.

Marijuana. The most commonly abused drug, marijuana is illegal except in a few states where it can be used for medicinal purposes. About 75 percent of Americans who use illegal drugs are marijuana users—an estimated 11 million people. Males ages 18–25 represent the largest users of marijuana, and about one in six men in this age group currently uses the drug. According to a 1999 national survey, 7.7 percent of youths ages 12–17 use marijuana at least once during the year.

Marijuana is far more potent now than in the past, so the drug has great potential for abuse and addiction. The use of marijuana also poses serious health consequences, such as memory loss, difficulty with problem solving and thinking, an increased heart rate, and problems with *anxiety* (see Volume 2) and panic attacks. Regular use of marijuana may lead to CANCERS.

Cocaine. About 1.5 million Americans use cocaine. Of these about 682,000 use the drug frequently, on 51 or more days a year. There are also an estimated 413,000 regular users of crack cocaine.

As with marijuana, cocaine is used mainly by individuals between the ages of 18–25, followed by adolescents ages 12–17. Men use the drug at about twice the rate of women. Cocaine usage also varies with race: the highest percentage of users are Hispanics, at 2.5 percent. Cocaine usage among African Americans and whites is about the same, at 1.9 and 1.7 percent.

Cocaine, particularly crack cocaine, is very addictive. There are also many health risks linked to abuse of the drug, including heart attack, respiratory failure, *stroke* (see Volume 8), and seizures. Those who inject cocaine and share needles risk contracting *sexually transmitted diseases (STDs)* (see Volumes 3, 7), including *HIV infections* (see Volume 7). Cocaine abuse can also cause severe psychological problems, including PSYCHOSIS.

Heroin. Heroin is a highly addictive illegal drug. A NARCOTIC, it is processed from morphine, a powerful painkiller. An estimated 200,000 people in the United States abuse heroin. Males are more likely to use the drug than females, and the largest group of heroin abusers is found among older users (over age 30). Numerous health risks are associated with the abuse of heroin, including the risk for HEART DISEASE and contracting HIV or viral HEPATITIS.

Amphetamines. Although AMPHETAMINES may be legally prescribed by physicians, the drugs are illegal when not prescribed. Also known as *speed* or *ice,* methamphetamine and other forms of amphetamines can produce an intense euphoria, or high. Amphetamine abuse can lead to heart problems, convulsions, and physical collapse. In some cases people die of amphetamine abuse. For example, methamphetamine is an extremely dangerous amphetamine involved in 501 deaths in the U.S. in 1998.

Inhalants. A variety of chemical products can be breathed in or inhaled to produce a high. About 883,000 people in the U.S. use INHALANTS, although it is difficult to determine the full extent of inhalant use because many substances legally sold in stores have the potential for abuse as inhalants. A number of inhalants are abused primarily by school-age children.

Substance Abuse in the U.S., 1998

Substance	Non-Hispanic White		Hispanic		African American	
	All Ages	Age 12–14	All Ages	Age 12–17	All Ages	Age 12–17
ALCOHOL	67.8	35.1	58.5	29.4	50.4	22.3
CIGARETTES	30.8	26.9	29.6	20.4	31.2	16.2
MARIJUANA	8.4	14.6	8.2	14.4	10.6	12.1
COCAINE	1.7	1.9	2.3	2.5	1.9	UNAVAIL.
INHALANTS	1.0	3.4	0.9	2.8	0.3	1.0
HEROIN	0.1	UNAVAIL.	0.1	UNAVAIL.	0.2	UNAVAIL.
ANY ILLEGAL DRUG	10.4	16.9	10.5	17.4	13.0	14.0

[Source: Substance Abuse and Mental Health Services Administration, *National Household Survey on Drug Abuse*, 1998.]

The use of inhalants carries a number of serious risks. Short-term effects from using these substances can include heart palpitations, dizziness, difficulty breathing, numbness in the hands and feet, and headaches. Prolonged or regular use of inhalants can have severe results such as damage to the kidneys, lungs, and liver; nausea and nosebleeds; loss of the sense of smell; damage to the nervous system; and irreversible brain damage. The drugs can also cause irregular heartbeat, severe mood swings, violent behavior, and death.

Harmful effects and death can occur with only one-time use of inhalants. Inhalants can kill in several different ways: First, sudden sniffing death syndrome may occur, usually as a result of cardiac arrest. Choking to death on one's own vomit is another risk. People who use inhalants can suffocate to death as a result of difficulty breathing. Users may also die from asphyxia, or the lack of oxygen, because fumes from the inhalants can decrease the breathable oxygen in the air to a level that makes it impossible to breathe. Likewise, death may result from *unintentional injuries* (see Volume 5) caused by careless behaviors that occur in association with inhaling the substances.

Hallucinogens. Hallucinogenic drugs include substances such as LSD and PCP that are known to produce vivid HALLUCINATIONS. Among the most typical abusers of these drugs are middle-class, suburban youths. The effects of some HALLUCINOGENS may last for as long as 12 hours. Chronic users of the drugs often need to take higher doses to reach the same level of euphoria. Taking higher doses is very dangerous, however, because the drugs can cause failure of the heart and lungs, convulsions, coma, and death. Use of hallucinogens can also result in serious psychological problems, including violent behavior, paranoia, *depression* (see Volume 2), and psychosis. In 1999 LSD was responsible for more than 5,000 emergency room visits in the United States.

Anabolic Steroids. ANABOLIC STEROIDS are most commonly abused by athletes and others who seek to increase the amount of muscle on their bodies or improve their athletic performance. Most users of these drugs are young adults. In 1997 about 1.8 percent of eighth graders and 2.4 percent of high school seniors in the U.S. had tried anabolic steroids at least once.

Use of anabolic steroids carries a number of serious risks. Men who abuse the drugs may suffer from impotence and have shrunken testicles. Women may develop masculine traits such as an increase in body hair, which is irreversible. The drugs can also cause violent rages and severe rashes. Other long-term effects of anabolic steroid abuse are heart disease, cancer, liver tumors, cataracts on the eyes, and death.

Designer Drugs. Sometimes called *club drugs*, these illegal substances are synthetic drugs derived from other drugs. Chronic use of designer drugs such as Ecstasy can cause brain damage or death. GHB, another dangerous designer drug, has caused at least 60 deaths in the United States.

According to a report from the National Institute of Drug Abuse, the use of club drugs in the United States has risen dramatically since 1999. The drugs are linked increasingly to cases of DRUG OVERDOSE and drug poisonings. Some of the substances are also used as DATE RAPE DRUGS.

Abuse of Prescription Drugs. Some people abuse drugs and medications prescribed either to themselves or to others. Among the prescribed drugs that may typically be abused are STIMULANTS such as Ritalin and certain BARBITURATES and painkillers.

Why People Abuse Drugs. Most people abuse drugs to achieve a feeling of euphoria or to escape personal problems. Many also find that the use of drugs helps to alleviate chronic pain, and this often leads to addiction. Addiction to prescribed medications often results from attempts to eliminate severe pain by taking higher than normal dosages of a drug and continuing its use beyond the prescribed period. Some people, especially adolescents, try drugs for the first time because of pressure from peers and friends. Ignoring the advice of others or their inner conscience, they comply with peer pressure because it seems easier than arguing about or flatly refusing to take the substance. Unfortunately, some drugs are very addictive, and people can become addicted after even one use. [*See also* ADDICTION AND PRESCRIPTION DRUGS; ADDICTION, CAUSES OF; DRUGS AND HEALTH PROBLEMS; PEER PRESSURE AND ADDICTION; TEENS AND ADDICTION].

DRUG ABUSE AND MENTAL HEALTH See Volume 2.

DRUG ADDICTION Psychological and physical dependence on a legal or ILLEGAL DRUG, which can lead to emotional and physical WITHDRAWAL symptoms if the substance is withheld. The most common addictive illegal drugs are HEROIN, COCAINE, and AMPHETAMINES. Among legal drugs TOBACCO is among the most addictive. Individuals may also have an ADDICTION to prescription drugs or even to some over-the-counter medications. Some 3.5 million Americans were addicted to illegal drugs in 1999.

Signs of drug addiction vary depending on the substance. Dilated (enlarged) pupils, for example, are a sign of cocaine or heroin addiction, while reddened eyes, increased appetite, and disorientation are symptoms of MARIJUANA abuse. Recent studies indicate that withdrawal from frequent use of marijuana may also cause aggressive behavior.

Drug addiction leads to a variety of social and health problems. Many addicts have little time for anything but using and getting more drugs, and thus they neglect school, work, and family. Additionally, long-term use of many drugs causes severe medical problems, from HIGH BLOOD PRESSURE to damage to the heart, kidneys, and other vital organs. Even one-time use of such drugs as ECSTASY, INHALANTS, or METHAMPHETAMINE can result in brain damage, seizures, coma, and death.

Treatment for drug addiction also depends on the drug. Heroin addicts, for example, are often treated with METHADONE. Addicts may need to undergo DETOXIFICATION in a rehabilitation facility, where they may receive medications to limit some of the more extreme symptoms associated with withdrawal. Many addicts benefit from counseling as well as from membership in a TWELVE-STEP PROGRAM such as Narcotics Anonymous or Cocaine Anonymous, both of which are modeled on ALCOHOLICS ANONYMOUS (AA). [See also DRUG ABUSE; DRUGS AND HEALTH PROBLEMS; DEPENDENCE, PHYSICAL; DEPENDENCE, PSYCHOLOGICAL; TOLERANCE, PHYSICAL.]

DRUG ENFORCEMENT ADMINISTRATION (DEA) Federal agency within the U.S. Department of Justice that enforces the laws on controlled substances, including legal and ILLEGAL DRUGS. The Drug Enforcement Administration, or DEA, investigates drug-related crimes, seizes property and money of drug dealers, and prosecutes drug cases in federal courts. It also works with state and local agencies involved in criminal matters related to drugs. Further, the DEA provides information on DRUG ABUSE for use in schools, communities, and other settings.

DRUG-FREE ZONES Areas set aside as specific places where no one may sell drugs. People selling any type of drugs in drug-free zones face harsher penalties than if they operate outside the zones. Generally aimed at protecting children and adolescents from drugs and drug dealing, drug-free zones are usually set up in and around schools or parks. [*See also* DRUG ABUSE; DRUG LAWS.]

DRUG INTERACTIONS The effects that result from taking two or more DRUGS (or ALCOHOL and one or more drugs) at the same time. Drug interactions can be potentially dangerous.

If an individual takes a combination of two or more drugs or a mixture of drugs and alcohol at the same time, each substance can change the effects of the other on the body. In some cases drug interactions can cause the action of one or more of the substances to be boosted or weakened. For example, if one particular drug causes an increase in blood pressure, the combination of another drug with it might further raise the blood pressure to dangerously high levels. A drug interaction can also cause effects that would not otherwise occur when taking drugs separately, such as extreme drowsiness.

Drug interactions can be very dangerous and even fatal. For example, when alcohol and COCAINE are both taken together, a new chemical substance called *cocaethylene* is created that is far more powerful than either the alcohol or cocaine taken alone. This particular drug interaction can cause death.

Drug interactions are not only a problem for illegal drug users or alcoholics. Anyone taking any medications should be aware that ingesting those drugs together with other medications, ILLEGAL DRUGS, or alcohol can also result in potentially dangerous drug interactions. [*See also* DRUG ABUSE; DRUG OVERDOSE; DRUGS AND HEALTH PROBLEMS.]

DRUG LAWS Federal and state laws aimed at controlling prescription medications, over-the-counter (OTC) drugs, and ILLEGAL DRUGS. The Food and Drug Administration (FDA) must approve nearly all new prescription and OTC medications before they may be sold to the American public. Drugs approved by the FDA have undergone extensive testing and have been proven not only safe but also effective. If any of these drugs are later found to cause medical problems, the FDA will withdraw them from the market. The FDA's control over drugs does not include herbal remedies, which fall under a special law for alternative medicines—the Dietary Supplement Health and Education Act.

Controlled Substances. Certain drugs that are considered to have a potential for abuse fall under the jurisdiction of a law known as the Controlled Substances Act and the supervision of the DRUG ENFORCEMENT ADMINISTRATION (DEA). The DEA classifies these **controlled substances**—both legal and illegal—into five categories known as schedules. These categories range from Schedule I (substances with the most potential for DRUG ABUSE and no accepted legal medical use) to Schedule V (drugs that may lead to some physical or psychological DEPENDENCE).

Among the drugs classified as Schedule I are HEROIN, LSD, MARIJUANA, HASHISH, and ECSTASY. Schedule II drugs include COCAINE, METHADONE, Ritalin, and the painkiller morphine. (Although cocaine is a highly addictive drug it does have some legal medical uses.) ANABOLIC STEROIDS are classified as Schedule III, while drugs such as Valium and Librium are included in Schedule IV. Drugs with codeine, such as the painkiller Tylenol 3 or certain cough syrups, are Schedule V drugs.

Laws on Drug Dealing and Possession. Individuals caught selling or buying illegal drugs may face serious criminal penalties, including time in jail. Generally, individuals considered to be drug dealers, or sellers of illegal drugs, are treated more harshly than the people who purchase the drugs. They also face federal laws against the sale of illegal drugs. However, people who buy drugs are also subject to both fines and jail time.

Even a first offense can bring a heavy fine and in some states the suspension of a driver's license for up to a year. In California first-time possession of marijuana can bring a fine of $100. In Indiana the fine for the same offense is $5,000. Some states also require individuals convicted of drug offenses to perform some type of community service. In Idaho, Indiana, and a number of other states it is considered a crime just to knowingly visit a place where drugs are used.

Individuals involved in drug offenses sometimes face more than fines and jail time. The DEA has the authority to seize any property involved with a crime involving illegal drugs. Thus, if a person used a car or boat to sell drugs, the DEA can confiscate the car or boat. The owner is not entitled to any compensation, nor can they get back their property. [*See also* DRUG-FREE ZONES.]

MORE SOURCES See www.ndsn.org

DRUG OVERDOSE Reaction of a body to an excessive amount of a drug. A drug overdose can cause ***stroke*** (see Volume 8), heart rhythm disorders, seizures, and sometimes psychotic behavior. It can also lead to coma and death.

Reasons for Overdose. People may accidentally overdose for several reasons. One reason may be that they inadvertently take too high a dose of a drug. In other cases the user may be unaware of dangerous DRUG INTERACTIONS that can occur when one drug is combined with another drug or ALCOHOL. Consuming alcohol and COCAINE at the same time, for example, can be fatal. People can also overdose by taking ILLEGAL DRUGS that contain unknown substances. Since the production of illegal drugs is not controlled, some drugs may sometimes contain various toxic chemicals and poisons. Besides accidental overdoses, individuals may purposely overdose on a drug while attempting *suicide* (see Volumes 2, 5). Suicidal drug overdoses often involve prescription medications such as BARBITURATES.

Effects of Overdose. The effects of a drug overdose depend on the substance ingested, the quantity taken, and other factors such as the weight of the victim and whether the person had eaten anything beforehand. Nevertheless, some generalizations can be made about overdoses with specific types of drugs.

An overdose of LSD generally results in more intense HALLUCINATIONS, PSYCHOSIS, and perhaps death. An overdose of MARIJUANA can also cause psychosis as well as paranoia, while overdoses of METHAMPHETAMINE often produce agitation, hallucinations, convulsions, and very high body temperature. A HEROIN overdose can result in shallow breathing, convulsions, coma, and death.

Treatment. Treatment for a drug overdose often involves pumping out the victim's stomach to remove some of the drug, as well as administering medications to treat the symptoms of the overdose. In order to treat the victim effectively, trained medical staff need as much information as possible, such as the drug taken, the dosage, and when the drug was taken. Anyone who discovers an individual who may have overdosed should take to the emergency room any medications or other drugs that may have been the source of the overdose. [*See also* DEATH FROM ADDICTIONS; DRUG ABUSE.]

DRUGS Chemicals that cause physical or psychological changes when introduced into the body. Legal medications are used to kill bacteria, decrease or end pain, limit symptoms of diseases, and provide **hormones** or other substances missing from a person's body or in short supply there. ILLEGAL DRUGS are generally used to create a feeling of euphoria or other heightened sensation. People with a DRUG ADDICTION also take the drugs to avoid the physical symptoms associated with WITHDRAWAL.

Legal drugs are either medications prescribed by physicians and dispensed by pharmacists or over-the-counter (OTC) drugs, which can be purchased without a prescription. Various alternative remedies, such as vitamin and mineral supplements and herbal substances, are also legal drugs. Although generally safe, legal drugs and alternative remedies can sometimes interact with ALCOHOL or other medications in ways that may be harmful. Some of these DRUG INTERACTIONS can even be life-threatening. There are also legal drugs, called **teratogens,** that are known to cause birth defects and should be avoided by pregnant women.

Illegal drugs cover a host of substances, including HEROIN, MARIJUANA, COCAINE, HASHISH, LSD, PCP, and various DESIGNER DRUGS such as ECSTASY. Possessing and selling these drugs are criminal offenses, and abuse of these substances can have very harmful effects on the health of the user.

Drugs can be swallowed, injected, or smoked. They can be dissolved under the tongue or inserted into the rectum. Some drugs also come on transdermal patches that are applied to the skin, which allows the drug to be absorbed more slowly into the bloodstream. A number of antismoking remedies used in NICOTINE REPLACEMENT THERAPY come in the form of transdermal patches.

All drugs have certain intended effects, whether to produce a feeling of euphoria in the case of various illegal drugs or to lower a fever or reduce inflammation in the case of certain prescription medications. Yet most drugs also produce side effects, which generally are unintended consequences of drug use. For example, an ANTIBIOTIC used to kill bacteria may also cause such side effects as stomach pain or diarrhea. An illegal drug taken to enhance mood may cause a dangerous rise in blood pressure or body temperature, as often occurs with drugs such as METHAMPHETAMINE.

Drug interactions are another problem to be considered by anyone using legal or illegal drugs. Taking one or more medications at the same time or mixing drugs with alcohol can result in dangerously heightened blood pressure and heart rate or can severely lower them. While some drug interactions can cause only temporary medical problems such as headaches or stomach aches, others can have more severe consequences, including coma and death. [*See also* ALCOHOL AND DRUGS, MOOD AND; DRUG ABUSE; DRUG OVERDOSE; DRUGS AND HEALTH PROBLEMS.]

DRUGS AND HEALTH PROBLEMS Medical problems caused by taking legal or ILLEGAL DRUGS. Most drugs that people take help treat ailments such as *diabetes mellitus, arthritis, infectious diseases* (see Volume 8), and other illnesses or health problems. Many other drugs, however, do not help the users. Instead, they may create health problems.

Illegal drugs such as HEROIN or CRACK COCAINE, or legal substances used in an illegal manner, such as INHALANTS, can be very harmful to health. Even prescribed drugs, when abused, can cause severe medical problems, including death. Some drugs may have short-term consequences or side effects that are rather mild, such as headaches or nausea. Others may have more moderate or serious effects as well as long-term consequences, such as damage to the heart, liver, or other organs in the body.

Among the factors that determine the effects of a drug on users are the length of time the drug has been taken and the dosage. The medical consequences of DRUG ABUSE also vary depending on the type of drug. For example, STIMULANTS can cause problems with the heart or the brain, while HEROIN can increase a person's risk of contracting serious infections such as *pneumonia* or *tuberculosis* (see Volume 8). For these reasons any discussion of the health problems associated with drugs must look at specific drugs or categories of drugs.

Heroin. Heroin users experience a euphoric high, which is the usual reason for the initial use of the drug. However, the drug also produces a number of undesirable short-term side effects, such as nausea, vomiting, and mental confusion. Pregnant women who use the drug may have a spontaneous abortion, or miscarriage.

Long-term use of heroin leads to severe ADDICTION as well as health problems such as collapsed veins from constant injections, infection of the heart and its valves, and the development of arthritic problems. Sharing needles or use of dirty needles increases the risk of contracting HIV, HEPATITIS, and other infectious diseases.

Cocaine. The short-term effects of COCAINE abuse include possible loss of the sense of smell, frequent nosebleeds, and constant runny noses. Users who inject the drug intravenously also risk contracting HIV or hepatitis. There are also short-term psychological consequences from cocaine use, including irritability, mood disturbances, paranoia, and episodes of uncontrollable rage. Cocaine users may also experience delusions and HALLUCINATIONS.

Among the long-term health consequences of cocaine use are addiction, frequent headaches, abdominal pain and nausea, an increased risk of heart attack or heart *arrhythmia* (see Volume 8), a risk of respiratory failure, and seizures.

Crack cocaine has its own risks. Besides the possibility of causing instant addiction, this form of cocaine has a number of short-term effects on health: dilated pupils, hyperthermia (a very high body temperature), HIGH BLOOD PRESSURE, and hyperactivity. These health consequences are heightened the longer the drug is used. Long-term crack use can lead to cardiac arrest or seizures.

Anabolic Steroids. ANABOLIC STEROIDS are drugs used illegally by some athletes who wish to bulk up, or add muscle. The short-term health consequences of using these drugs can include severe acne and high blood pressure. Men who continue abusing anabolic steroids may experience hair loss, impotence, and breast development.

Although steroids are used primarily by men, some women also use the drugs to increase their muscular strength. Women who abuse anabolic steroids may develop masculine characteristics such as an increased growth of body hair and decreased breast size.

The long-term health consequences of steroid use for both men and women include impaired fertility, damage to the heart and liver, and severe psychiatric problems.

Hallucinogens. Hallucinogenic drugs may cause a person to feel powerful or to experience a feeling of euphoria. Short-term or long-term use may also cause HALLUCINATIONS and paranoia. Long after HALLUCINOGENS are out of the body's system, users may experience **flashbacks**.

Long-term effects of hallucinogenic drugs can include coma and death. Serious injury is also a possibility, since the drugs severely impair a person's judgment. For example, users may think they are invulnerable and will jump off high buildings or take other risky actions they would not normally pursue.

Inhalants. Even a one-time use of an inhalant may cause severe medical harm, such as damage to the brain and lungs or death. Short-term health problems associated with use of these drugs include headaches, vomiting, and mental confusion. Long-term use of inhalants can lead to kidney damage, liver damage, hearing loss, and brain damage.

Amphetamines. AMPHETAMINES raise the blood pressure and pulse rates of users and may provide a short-term feeling of euphoria. The short-term or long-term health problems associated with the drugs include heavy sweating, impaired muscle coordination, insomnia, *anorexia* (see Volume 4), blurred vision, and physical and mental collapse. Use of the drugs also has psychological consequences such as delusions and paranoia. Amphetamine abusers also may exhibit violent behavior; and the longer the drug is used, the more likely the individual will become violent.

Methamphetamine. METHAMPHETAMINE can produce serious health consequences. The short-term effects of these synthetic stimulants include euphoria, agitation, and increased respiration. Another short-term reaction to the drugs is hyperthermia, or very high body temperatures, which can lead to death. Methamphetamine abuse has a number of serious long-term health consequences, including convulsions, memory loss, brain damage, heart damage, mental confusion, motion disorders that mimic *Parkinson's disease* (see Volume 8), hallucinations, paranoia, heart attack, *stroke* (see Volume 8), and PSYCHOSIS.

Marijuana or Hashish. The short-term effect of using marijuana or hashish only a few times is generally a feeling of euphoria and disorientation. Regular users of these drugs, however, may experience such health problems as memory loss, difficulty with problem solving and thinking, increased heart rate, *anxiety,* and *panic disorder* (see Volume 2). As with cigarette use, long-term regular use of marijuana is associated with respiratory problems, including BRONCHITIS and *pneumonia* (see Volume 8). Some experts believe that long-term exposure to marijuana may also lead to the development of CANCERS.

DRUG TESTING Testing of a body fluid, usually blood or urine, to detect the presence of ILLEGAL DRUGS or ALCOHOL in the body. Drug testing is usually done to screen for MARIJUANA, COCAINE, HEROIN, or alcohol, but athletic organizations may also test for ANABOLIC STEROIDS or AMPHETAMINES. There are various ways to test for drugs, but the most common is probably urine testing, or urinalysis. Occasionally, blood testing will be done instead of or in addition to urinalysis.

Some employers require drug testing before they will hire an individual and check for those using drugs at regular intervals. States may require that people in certain professions, such as those working with children, be cleared through drug testing before being hired.

People who operate heavy or dangerous equipment or who are responsible for the safety of others (such as pilots) may be screened routinely for drugs. Prisoners or individuals on parole or probation may also be subjected to drug testing. Testing is done regularly on athletes, and those who test positive for drugs are disqualified from participating in athletic events. Government agencies may require drug-screening tests of employees, and military organizations may have random drug testing of service personnel.

People suspected of DRIVING WHILE INTOXICATED OR DRUG IMPAIRED may be required by state law to undergo testing for alcohol to determine whether BLOOD ALCOHOL LEVELS exceed the legal limits for INTOXICATION. Drivers may be given the choice of either a urine test, blood test, or a test by a device called a Breathalyzer, which detects alcohol on a person's breath.

Drug testing can be very valuable. People found to be addicted to drugs or alcohol can be removed from positions in which they could put the health and safety of others at risk. Testing also identifies abusers so they can be treated for their ADDICTION.

DRUG USE See DRUG ABUSE.

DRUG WITHDRAWAL See DRUG ADDICTION; WITHDRAWAL.

DRUNKENNESS See INTOXICATION.

ECSTASY Popular and ILLEGAL DRUG often associated with night life, discos, and RAVES; also known by other names such as Adam, Cloud Nine, Eve, and Essence. Ecstasy is a STIMULANT that is usually available in a tablet or capsule, although the drug can be injected. A synthetic drug derived from a METHAMPHETAMINE, Ecstasy is the street name for MDMA (methylenedioxymethamphetamine).

One of the most popular so-called DESIGNER DRUGS or CLUB DRUGS, Ecstasy was first developed in 1914 as a diet drug. It was later withdrawn from the market because of severe side effects. The drug resurfaced in the mid-1990s and became popular with young adults. Use of the drug among teens increased from 5 percent in 1995 to about 10 percent by the year 2000.

Users of Ecstasy say that the drug causes profoundly positive feelings, empathy for others, reduction of *anxiety* (see Volume 2), and extreme relaxation. The drug also suppresses the need to eat or sleep, thus allowing users to stay up all day and night, sometimes remaining awake for 2–3 days. Most users are adolescents and young adults who like the idea of avoiding food and sleep to concentrate on partying. They also believe the drug will give them a sexual high, although there is no evidence that Ecstasy enhances sexual experiences.

The effects of Ecstasy can last for 24 hours, and side effects may linger for weeks or longer. Some of these side effects include dehydration, HIGH BLOOD PRESSURE, *depression* (see Volume 2), delusions of persecution, confusion, *sleep disorders* (see Volumes 2, 8), panic attacks, and anxiety. Ecstasy may also cause *stroke* (see Volume 8), kidney failure, seizures, heart attack, and tremors. Jaw clenching and teeth grinding are also common side effects of the drug, and some users suck on baby pacifiers to relieve some of the tension that this produces.

What about Ecstasy?

Although many teens report that they know Ecstasy is a dangerous drug, the use of this drug continues to rise among young people. Many adolescents may believe that it is safe to experiment with the drug once or twice and that, as long as they are not a regular user, they cannot really get hurt.

Adolescents who believe that are putting themselves in grave risk. Ecstasy can cause brain damage and even death at any time—the first time an individual tries the drug may be the last time they try it. This drug is not worth the risk of brain damage or death, so stay away from it.

Ecstasy is known to cause hyperthermia in some people, which is a dangerous and sometimes fatal increase in body temperature. Some rave clubs provide cold showers to help attendees on Ecstasy bring down their body temperatures. Strong evidence also suggests that Ecstasy can cause permanent brain damage. Brain scans performed on people and animals by the National Institute of Mental Health have found brain changes that impair learning and memory—changes that may be permanent. While Ecstasy is dangerous for everyone, it is especially risky for those with high blood pressure, liver disease, or heart problems.

EMPHYSEMA A very serious and incurable *lung disease* (see Volume 8) characterized by oversized and damaged air sacs (called *alveoli*) in the lungs. This damage to the lungs causes difficulty breathing and a chronic severe cough. Those with *emphysema* may also suffer from chronic BRONCHITIS and are a greater risk of getting a lung infection like *pneumonia* (see Volume 8).

The shortness of breath and severe coughing of emphysema become increasingly worse and usually lead to HEART DISEASE. The disease eventually becomes debilitating, and people with advanced emphysema must take oxygen to help breathing. Emphysema is usually fatal, and death comes from either heart failure or the inability to breathe at all.

Emphysema usually develops as a result of years of smoking TOBACCO products. Hereditary factors may also be involved. Over 1 million Americans are afflicted with emphysema, and about 18,000 die each year from the disease.

EPIDEMIOLOGY Study of the distribution of and factors that cause diseases and other health problems in groups of people. It is epidemiologists—scientists who are experts in epidemiology—who usually discover the causes behind specific types of diseases, injuries, and medical conditions.

Epidemiologists conduct studies that involve making observations and collecting data on many people who may have been, or who may be, victims of substance abuse or addiction. Sometimes an epidemiological study may deal with something as simple as trying to determine the mortality or death rate associated with a type of disease among a specific group or population—for instance, how many people between ages 18 and 21 die as a result of drug or alcohol overdose.

More often, epidemiological studies involve searching for complex links or connections between diseases and other factors. Scientists who conduct such studies, for example, may discover that many pregnant women who smoke deliver low-birthweight babies.

This finding becomes a strong clue, although not proof, that smoking may be linked to low birthweight. A study like this would then lead to more research. The study may be repeated to make sure that no errors in observations or in the collection of data were made, and similar studies may be conducted to look more closely at the links between smoking and low birthweight. If enough epidemiological studies achieve the same results, and the association between smoking and low birthweight is strong and consistent, scientists may conclude that smoking is not just associated with low birthweight, but may cause it. Such an understanding may lead to better ways of prevention. [*See also* PREGNANCY AND TOBACCO, ALCOHOL, AND DRUGS.]

F

FETAL ALCOHOL SYNDROME (FAS) A type of birth defect that affects as many as 12,000 children in the United States each year. Fetal alcohol syndrome occurs in children born to women who abused ALCOHOL during *pregnancy* (see Volume 3). Children with FAS are often born prematurely. Most have low birthweights and small head circumferences, and they may continue to be small for their age as they grow older.

Children with FAS often have characteristic facial features, including short noses, small chins, and a general flattened facial appearance. Because these features are often not apparent until the child grows older, many children with FAS are not diagnosed until they are about six years old or older.

Children with FAS often have a variety of medical problems, including *cerebral palsy* (see Volume 8) and seizures. They may also have learning disabilities, attention deficit disorders, and mental retardation. About a third of children with FAS have heart defects. Children with FAS may also have cleft palates, kidney problems, and hernias.

Doctors recommend that all women who are pregnant—or women who even think that they may be pregnant or would like to become pregnant—should avoid alcohol use during their pregnancy. While drinking alcohol during any part of the pregnancy is potentially harmful to the developing fetus, drinking during the first three months is particularly harmful. [*See also* PREGNANCY AND TOBACCO, ALCOHOL, AND DRUGS.]

FREEBASING A method used to convert COCAINE into CRACK COCAINE so that it can be smoked. In freebasing, cocaine is heated with a flammable fluid such as ether. This process concentrates the drug, which is then smoked in a pipe or a cigarette containing MARIJUANA. The effects of the crack cocaine are felt within seconds, and the drug is very addicting.

HALLUCINATIONS Sensory experiences in which a person sees, hears, or feels things that are not really there. For example, people experiencing hallucinations may see changing colors or shapes, hear voices talking to them from a newspaper, smell some odor that is not really present, or feel bugs crawling inside their skin.

People with a *mental illness* such as *schizophrenia* (see Volume 2) or who suffer from a brain disorder such as *Alzheimer's disease* (see Volume 8) may experience hallucinations. Individuals who are not mentally ill may hallucinate as a result of taking HALLUCINO-GENS such as LSD or as a consequence of long-term ALCOHOL ABUSE. People undergoing alcohol WITHDRAWAL and suffering from DELIRIUM TREMENS (DTs) often experience a variety of hallucinations. Very high doses of painkilling OPIATES such as morphine may also cause people to hallucinate.

Hallucinations can be extremely terrifying experiences. They can also be very dangerous. If people act on the basis of a hallucination, they may cause serious harm to themselves or to others. For example, a person who feels bugs crawling under their skin may scratch deeply or cut themselves to try to remove them. An individual trying to escape from a hallucinated monster could run into traffic and be killed.

HALLUCINOGENS Drugs that can produce elevated moods, unusual sensations, and HALLUCINATIONS of sights, sounds, or smells that are not really present. LSD, MESCALINE, and PCP (phenylcyclo-hexyl) are all hallucinogens, as are some DESIGNER DRUGS such as

Commonly Abused Drugs: Hallucinogens

Substances	Examples of Proprietary or Street Names	Medical Uses	Route of Administration	DEA Schedules*	Period of Detection
LSD	Acid, Microdot	None	Oral	I	8 hours
Mescaline	Buttons, Cactus, Mesc, Peyote	None	Oral	I	2–3 days
Phencyclidine and Analogs	PCP; Angel Dust, Boat, Hog, Love Boat	Anesthetic (veterinary)	Injected, oral, smoked	I, II	2–8 days
Psilocybin	Magic Mushroom, Purple Passion, Shrooms	None	Oral	I	8 hours
Amphetamine variants	DOB, DOM, MDA, MDMA; Adam, Ecstasy, STP, XTC	None	Oral	I	1–2 days
Marijuana	Blunt, Grass, Herb, Pot, Reefer, Sinsemilla, Smoke, Weed	None	Oral, smoked	I	1 day–5 weeks
Hashish	Hash	None	Oral, smoked	I	1 day–5 weeks
Tetrahydrocannabinol	Marinol, THC	Antiemetic	Oral, smoked	I, II	1 day–5 weeks
Anabolic Steriods	Testosterone (T/E ration), Stanazolol, Nandroiene	Hormone Replacement Therapy	Oral, Injected	III	Oral; up to 3 weeks (for testosterone and others); Injected: up to 3 months (Nandrolene up to 9 months)

*Drug Enforcement Administration (DEA) Schedule I and II drugs have a high potential for abuse. They require greater security and have a quota on manufacture, among other restrictions. Schedule I drugs are available for research only and have no approved medical use. Schedule II drugs are available only through prescription, cannot have refills, and require a form for ordering. Schedule III drugs are available with prescription, may have five refills in six months, and may be ordered verbally.

[Source: National Institue on Drug Abuse, *Sixth Annual Report to Congress,* 2001.]

ECSTASY. Some hallucinogens are natural substances; others are synthetic. For example, mescaline is derived from the juice of the peyote cactus, while PCP and Ecstasy are synthetically created from chemicals.

Hallucinogens may cause a person to see, hear, smell, or feel things that are not really there—sensations known as hallucinations. For example, users may hallucinate that snakes are crawling all over the floor or that they hear voices coming from a newspaper. The sensory distortions in hallucinations may cause users to see objects as extremely large or much smaller than they are. All of these sensations and feelings are very real to the individual experiencing the hallucination.

Some individuals who have taken hallucinogens have been severely injured or have died while under the influence of the drugs because they believed they could fly or perform other impossible feats. Attempting such deeds can cause serious injury or death. Hallucinogens often create mental confusion, and they can also cause convulsions, coma, and death. Some of the drugs are also known for their flashback effect, in which a person may experience hallucinations long after the drug is out of the body's system.

HASHISH An ILLEGAL DRUG made from the resin of the flowers and leaves of the hemp plant (known scientifically as *Cannabis sativa*) and usually smoked. The effects of hashish—which include exaggerated sensations and a feeling of euphoria—are similar to those of MARIJUANA, although hashish may be much stronger. Both hashish and marijuana contain an active chemical ingredient called THC (tetrahydrocannabinol), which causes some of the drugs' intoxicating effects.

HEART DISEASE Disease of the heart or its valves. The abuse of TOBACCO, DRUGS, or ALCOHOL can be harmful to the heart and contribute to *coronary heart disease* (see Volume 8).

Smoking stresses the heart and the blood vessels and can lead to chronic heart disease or heart attack. It also increases blood pressure, furthering the risk for damage to the heart. Abuse of various DRUGS can also cause serious damage to the heart and can lead to heart attack and death.

ALCOHOL ABUSE can harm the heart by causing it to enlarge. Heavy drinking may also diminish the ability of the heart to contract, a condition called *alcoholic cardiomyopathy*. One symptom of this condition is shortness of breath. Alcohol abuse can also result in high blood pressure, heart attack, and irregular heart rhythms, or *arrhythmia* (see Volume 8), which may lead to death. [*See also* ALCOHOL AND HEALTH PROBLEMS; TOBACCO AND HEALTH PROBLEMS.]

HELP—911 A special phone number for use in emergencies. In most parts of the United States, calling 911 in the event of an emergency will rapidly summon emergency medical staff or a police officer directly to your home. Use of this number can and does save the lives of people facing health crises resulting from the abuse of DRUGS or ALCOHOL. People addicted to drugs or alcohol are more likely to experience severe medical problems that require emergency attention, such as a DRUG OVERDOSE, DELIRIUM TREMENS, or ALCOHOL POISONING. If individuals are too ill or intoxicated to obtain such assistance on their own, others may need to call 911 and contact emergency personnel on their behalf.

HEPATITIS An inflammation of the liver that can be caused by a virus or by ALCOHOL ABUSE. The viral form of *hepatitis* (see Volume 8) is often found among people who heavily abuse DRUGS and share dirty needles to inject HEROIN, COCAINE, or other drugs intravenously. Alcoholic hepatitis is caused by many years of severe ALCOHOLISM that has caused permanent liver disease. In the most advanced stages of the disease hepatitis can cause death. [*See also* ALCOHOL AND HEALTH PROBLEMS.]

HEROIN An extremely addicting ILLEGAL DRUG derived from the opium poppy. Heroin may be smoked, snorted (inhaled), or injected directly into the bloodstream. Injecting the drug can be very dangerous because of the possibility of contracting HIV from contaminated needles.

Heroin abuse is a growing problem in the United States. According to the DRUG ENFORCEMENT ADMINISTRATION (DEA), the number of heroin users in the nation rose from 68,000 in 1993 to 208,000 in 1999. At the same time, the average age of heroin users has dropped. In 1995 the average age of first-time heroin users was 25, but by 1998 this figure fell to age 21. Meanwhile, heroin deaths have increased in recent years. In Florida, for example, heroin-related deaths rose from 28 in 1993 to 206 in 1998.

Effects of Heroin. Heroin causes a state of euphoria, sleepiness, nausea, and constricted pupils in the eyes. These effects do not reflect the great dangers of the drug and the severe health consequences that it can have on users. Today, heroin is even more dangerous than in the past because the potency of the drug is greater now than in past years.

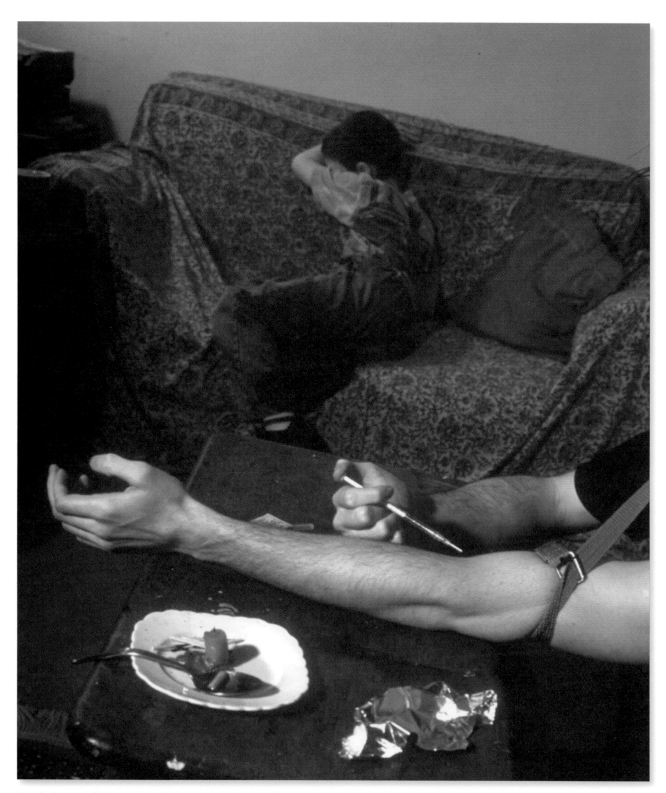

Heroin is one of the most addictive and dangerous illegal drugs.

An overdose of heroin can slow breathing and cause convulsions, coma, and death. Heroin users are also at greater risk for getting *bacterial infections* (see Volume 8), especially of the liver and kidneys. Other common diseases among heroin addicts are *pneumonia* and *tuberculosis* (see Volume 8). Heroin addicts are more susceptible to these two diseases partly because they are in poor health and also because heroin depresses respiration.

Addictive substances often found in street heroin may clog the blood vessels leading to the liver, kidneys, lungs, or brain, and this can cause serious infection. In addition, the sharing of needles between drug addicts can transmit HEPATITIS, HIV, or other *sexually transmitted diseases (STDs)* (see Volume 7).

Heroin Withdrawal. Heroin is highly addictive, and the addict needs greater and greater amounts of the drug to achieve the same effect as in the past. When users stop taking the drug, they experience various physical symptoms upon WITHDRAWAL, including severe muscle and bone pain, vomiting, diarrhea, and involuntary leg movements. Because the withdrawal symptoms are so severe, heroin addicts seek more heroin to avoid them. Withdrawal symptoms reach a peak from 24 to 48 hours after the last dose of heroin is taken, and they continue for about a week. Because of the severity of withdrawal and the difficulty in stopping use of the drug, experts recommend that heroin addicts undergoes DETOXIFICATION in a hospital or rehabilitation program designed to treat ADDICTION.

Treatment for Heroin Addiction. Heroin addicts frequently require treatment in a residential treatment program where they will live for a minimum of three to six months. Some medications, such as METHADONE or LAAM (levo-alpha-acetyl-methadol), have proven effective in helping addicts reduce their drug habit. Therapy may also enable heroin addicts to end their addiction permanently. [*See also* DRUGS AND HEALTH PROBLEMS.]

HIGH BLOOD PRESSURE An elevated level of blood pressure against the walls of arteries; also known as *hypertension*. Smoking, heavy alcohol use, and the abuse of many drugs can lead to the development or worsening of *high blood pressure* (see Volume 8). Among the drugs that can cause an increase in blood pressure are AMPHETAMINES, ANABOLIC STEROIDS, COCAINE, CRACK COCAINE, ECSTASY, and METHAMPHETAMINE. Since many people who smoke or take drugs also drink alcohol, the combined factors increase the risk for hypertension. High blood pressure can lead to serious health problems, including HEART DISEASE, kidney disease, and *stroke* (see Volume 8). [*See also* ALCOHOL AND HEALTH PROBLEMS.]

HIV The virus that causes acquired immune deficiency syndrome, or *AIDS* (see Volume 7). People who abuse drugs have an increased risk for developing HIV. There are several reasons for this. One reason is that drug abusers often share contaminated needles to inject HEROIN, COCAINE, or other drugs. In doing so, they may exchange body fluids that contain the infectious agents that cause HIV as well as other diseases such as HEPATITIS and *sexually transmitted diseases (STDs)* like *syphilis* or *gonorrhea* (see Volumes 3, 7).

Another reason for the increased risk of HIV among drug abusers is that they are more likely to engage in unsafe sex. While in a drugged or intoxicated state, drug users are more likely to engage in sex with multiple partners and to have sex without using condoms. Both of these actions are risk factors for the spread of HIV as well as other sexually transmitted diseases. Drug abusers—as well as alcoholics—may also be more susceptible to contracting HIV because they are in a weakened condition of health, although this relationship has not been proven.

Studies of drug abusers indicate that the risk of contracting HIV may be greatly reduced by participation in a treatment program. According to the National Institute on Drug Abuse, injection-drug users who do not enter treatment are six times more likely to become infected with HIV than those who enter and complete a course of treatment. [*See also* ALCOHOL AND DRUGS, SEX AND; DRUGS AND HEALTH PROBLEMS.]

HUFFING The practice of sniffing or inhaling products for the purpose of attaining an artificial high. Huffing is an extremely dangerous practice that can cause permanent brain damage and death, even after just one time. There are over a thousand household products that can be abused as INHALANTS, including paint thinners, gasoline, glue, room fresheners, and various products in aerosol cans. Most abusers of these products are adolescent boys, usually in junior high school. Since 1996 at least 270 teenagers in the United States have died as a result of huffing.

HYPNOTHERAPY A form of therapy that induces a light trancelike state. People undergoing hypnotherapy are first put in a trancelike state of *hypnosis* (see Volume 2). While in this hypnotic state, the individuals are given suggestions to change certain behaviors, such as quitting smoking, eating less, or exercising more. A trained hypnotherapist may be fairly successful in helping a person limit addicting behaviors. However, other therapies or methods are often needed as well, including use of medications or membership in a self-help group such as ALCOHOLICS ANONYMOUS (AA). Some individuals may be successful in learning self-hypnosis so that they can continue on their own to work at ending addicting behaviors.

ILLEGAL DRUGS Drugs that are against the law to possess, sell, or use. The term *illegal drugs* generally refers to such substances as HEROIN, MARIJUANA, COCAINE, CRACK COCAINE, and LSD. While it is also illegal to use prescription drugs that are prescribed for others, these are generally not considered illegal drugs.

People use illegal drugs to attain some sort of a high, which may involve feelings of **euphoria,** extreme relaxation, or HALLUCINATIONS. However, use of these drugs can also cause many serious health problems, including heart failure, seizures, coma, and even death. In addition, illegal drugs cause people to lose their inhibitions, making it more likely that they may engage in behaviors that could endanger their safety or health, such as participating in unsafe sex or DRIVING WHILE INTOXICATED OR DRUG IMPAIRED.

Local, state, and federal law enforcement agencies, as well as federal organizations such as the DRUG ENFORCEMENT ADMINISTRATION (DEA), have the authority to arrest people who possess illegal drugs or sell them to others. Punishments for the possession or sale of illegal drugs may involve jail time as well as fines and the confiscation of property.

School authorities also have authority to punish students who bring illegal drugs to public or private schools. Schools often have policies that automatically expel any student found with drugs. Many schools are also part of so-called DRUG-FREE ZONES in which the penalties for drug dealing are harsher than they are in areas outside the zones. These special zones are aimed at protecting children and adolescents from illegal drugs. [*See also* DRUG ABUSE; DRUG ADDICTION.]

Keywords

euphoria an exaggerated feeling of well-being that has no basis in reality.

INHALANTS Drugs that produce an artificial high by breathing in or inhaling them. There are hundreds of different substances that can be inhaled to produce a high. These so-called inhalants include a number of common household products such as paints, glues, and air fresheners. Abuse of these substances generally involves inhaling the fumes they give off, which produces an artificial high for the user. Most abusers of inhalants are adolescents, particularly boys.

A few prescription inhalant drugs are also abused, such as AMYL NITRATE, a drug used to treat patients with heart disease. Abuse of amyl nitrate, which some people mistakenly believe will enhance a sexual experience, can cause unconsciousness, heart attack, or even death.

Inhalant abuse is very dangerous because it can cause brain damage and death even with first-time use. Health problems associated with inhaling paint fumes, solvents, and various other inhalants include damage to the heart, kidney, liver, and brain, as well as hearing loss. Inhalant abusers also may experience problems such as headache, vomiting, and mental confusion. Some substances that are inhaled may cause *leukemia* (see Volume 8). [*See also* DRUG ABUSE; DRUGS AND HEALTH PROBLEMS.]

INJECTIONS Taking drugs directly into the bloodstream or a muscle by an injection with a hypodermic needle or syringe. People regularly receive injections of prescription drugs to protect themselves against diseases such as HEPATITIS, *tetanus,* and *diphtheria* (see Volume 8) or to treat ailments such as *diabetes mellitus* (see Volume 8). Some drug abusers also inject ILLEGAL DRUGS, including HEROIN and COCAINE. With illegal drugs injections allow the drugs to take effect much faster than with other methods, which is usually the reason why many drug abusers choose injections over smoking or inhaling the drug or taking it in pill form. Some drug abusers have heavily scarred arms or legs or severe scars on other parts of their bodies as a result of numerous injections they take. Injecting illegal drugs can also increase the risk of contracting infections such as hepatitis, *HIV infections,* and other *sexually transmitted diseases (STDs)* (see Volume 7). [*See also* DRUGS AND HEALTH PROBLEMS; INTRAVENOUS USE OF ILLEGAL DRUGS.]

INTOXICATION Also known as *drunkenness,* an impaired physical and mental state that occurs as a result of excessive consumption of ALCOHOL. Typical symptoms of intoxication include slurred or confused speech; uncoordinated body movements; and extreme or inappropriate emotions, such as crying or laughing hysterically.

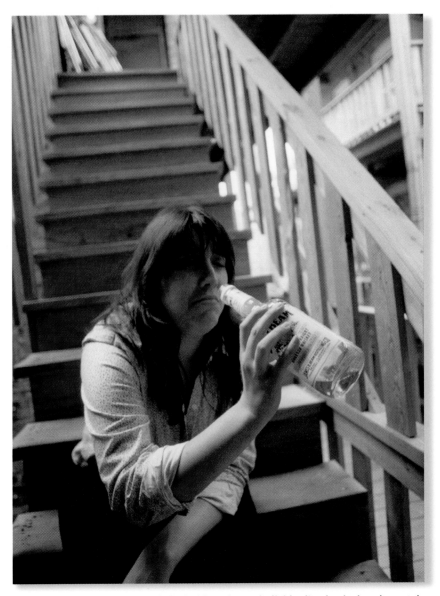

The excessive consumption of alcohol impairs an individual's physical and mental abilities.

In most cases the degree of intoxication decreases as the body absorbs the alcohol. Sometimes, however, people consume so much alcohol over such a short period of time that their bodies cannot absorb the alcohol quickly enough. This puts them at risk of ALCOHOL POISONING, which can be fatal. The risk of alcohol poisoning is especially high in instances of BINGE DRINKING.

Intoxication can be measured in terms of BLOOD ALCOHOL LEVELS. Each state in the U.S. has set a particular blood alcohol level as a limit of legal intoxication. People who test over that limit are considered legally drunk. In addition, ZERO TOLERANCE LAWS have established especially low blood alcohol levels as the limit of legal intoxication for drivers under age 21. These levels differ depending on the state. [*See also* ALCOHOL ABUSE; ALCOHOL LAWS.]

INTRAVENOUS USE OF ILLEGAL DRUGS INJECTIONS of an ILLEGAL DRUG directly into a vein. Some drug abusers prefer intravenous drug use because this method allows the drugs to take effect faster than with other methods. Among the drugs most commonly injected intravenously are HEROIN, COCAINE and METHAMPHETAMINE.

Intravenous drug use is very dangerous. For one thing, users may be careless and harm themselves while doing the injection. For example, they might mistakenly hit an artery instead of a vein, causing them to bleed profusely. An even greater danger is the risk of infection. Intravenous drug users often share needles, and dirty or contaminated needles can transmit **HIV infections** (see Volume 7), HEPATITIS, and other infections, including *sexually transmitted diseases (STDs)* (see Volume 7). [*See also* DRUG ABUSE; DRUG ADDICTION; DRUGS AND HEALTH PROBLEMS.]

IV DRUG USE See INTRAVENOUS USE OF ILLEGAL DRUGS.

LEADING CAUSES OF DEATH FROM ADDICTIONS See DEATH FROM ADDICTIONS.

LIQUOR See ALCOHOL.

LSD A potent HALLUCINOGEN. An ILLEGAL DRUG, LSD (lysergic acid diethylamide) is generally found in tablet form, often in tiny pills called *microdots*. The drug may also be placed on sugar cubes or on tiny pieces of paper. The effects of the drug can last for as long as 10–12 hours.

People who take LSD often experience euphoria and disorientation. Other effects of the drug include profuse sweating, dilation of the pupils of the eyes, nausea, extreme mood changes, a distorted sense of time, a rapid heart rate, and a drop in body temperature. Users often have various types of HALLUCINATIONS; for example, objects may appear distorted or colors seem unusually vibrant. They may experience synesthesia, a blending of the senses in which a person "hears" colors or "sees" sounds. LSD may also induce paranoia, an irrational fear of persecution by others. One unique feature of LSD is that a person may suffer flashbacks— sudden recurrences of sensory distortions and other hallucinations that may occur days, months, or even several years after taking the drug.

LSD is a dangerous drug primarily because of its psychological effects. Some people who take the drug experience so-called "bad trips," which may include perceptions of monsters, extreme delusions, and severe panic. Some LSD users have been known to perform violent acts or to act in ways that may harm themselves or others. For example, individuals under the influence of LSD may think that they can fly and jump off a building. The drug can also trigger serious *depression* (see Volume 2) and PSYCHOSIS. [*See also* DRUGS AND HEALTH PROBLEMS.]

LUNG CANCER Cancer of the lung tissues. The leading cause of death from cancer in the United States, *lung cancer* (see Volume 8) represents about 28 percent of all cancer deaths. In 1999 about 160,000 Americans died from this disease. Ninety percent of lung cancer deaths are attributed to the regular use of TOBACCO.

Tobacco and Lung Cancer. Although lung cancer can develop from a variety of causes, research indicates that the overwhelming number of cases results from smoking cigarettes, cigars, or pipes. The risk for smokers developing lung cancer depends on such factors as when they started smoking, how many years they have smoked, and how many cigarettes they smoke daily. Another risk factor is how deeply tobacco smoke is inhaled. Inhaling tobacco smoke deeply into the lungs increases the risk for developing lung cancer. In general, heavy smokers and people who began smoking as children or adolescents and continue smoking throughout adulthood have the greatest risk for developing the disease.

Symptoms and Treatment. Among the common symptoms of lung cancer are a persistent cough that does not get better, coughing up of blood, frequent infections of BRONCHITIS or *pneumonia* (see Volume 8), swelling in the face and neck, hoarseness, and feeling short of breath or constantly tired.

The treatment for lung cancer depends on how far the disease has advanced. Patients generally receive chemotherapy with

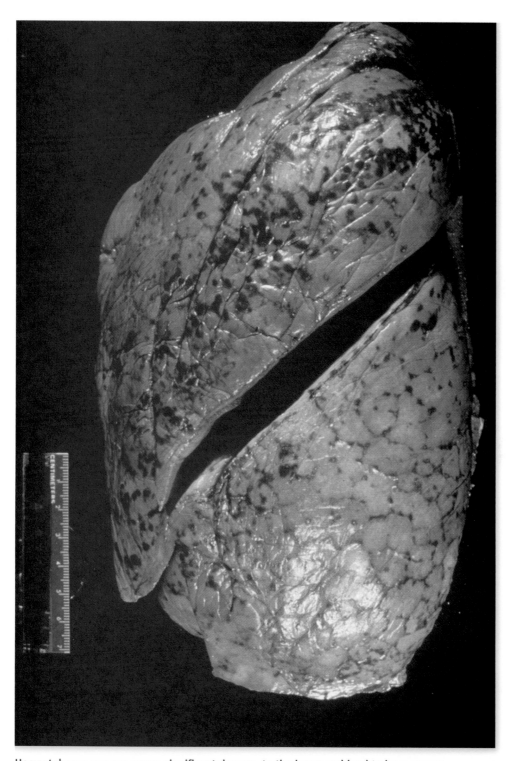

Heavy tobacco use can cause significant damage to the lungs and lead to lung cancer.

anticancer drugs to destroy cancer cells. They may also have surgery, which may include removal of a lung, followed by additional chemotherapy.

Radiation therapy, another form of treatment for lung cancer, uses high-energy rays to destroy the cancer cells. It may also be used to treat symptoms such as shortness of breath. Sometimes a special form of laser therapy, called photodynamic therapy, is used to treat small tumors in the lungs. [*See also* TOBACCO AND HEALTH PROBLEMS.]

MAINLINING Term sometimes used for the direct injection of an ILLEGAL DRUG into a major blood vessel. Among the drugs most commonly mainlined are HEROIN and COCAINE. When a drug is injected by mainlining, its effects occur within seconds rather than the minutes it would take if the drug were smoked or ingested orally. If mainlining is performed too often on the same blood vessels, those blood vessels may eventually collapse. Mainlining can be very dangerous. A careless or impaired drug user could hit an artery, causing uncontrollable bleeding. If the bleeding is not stopped, the user could die from loss of blood before help arrives. Mainlining can also increase the risk of infection if users share needles or the needles used are dirty or contaminated. Among the infections that can be transmitted by injection drug use are HEPATITIS, *HIV infections* (see Volume 7), and *sexually transmitted diseases (STDs)* (see Volumes 3, 7). [*See also* INJECTIONS; INTRAVENOUS USE OF ILLEGAL DRUGS.]

MARIJUANA A drug that comes from the stems, leaves, and flowering tops of the *Cannabis sativa* plant. Also known by various street names such as grass, pot, and weed, marijuana is the most commonly abused ILLEGAL DRUG in the United States. About 75 percent of all illegal drug abusers are marijuana users. In 1999 about 2 million Americans of all ages used marijuana or HASHISH, another drug that comes from the cannabis plant. Most marijuana users are males between the ages of 18 and 25.

Effects of Marijuana. Marijuana is usually smoked in a cigarette-like form called a *joint* or in hollowed-out cigars called *blunts*. Some abusers add other drugs, such as PCP, to their marijuana to produce heightened effects.

Marijuana is rapidly absorbed into the body and may generate feelings of disorientation and euphoria. The drug also produces some of the same effects as certain HALLUCINOGENS—heightened sensitivity to colors and sounds, sensory distortion, and a distorted sense of time—but marijuana is generally much less potent.

Frequent use of marijuana can have severe consequences, resulting in learning disabilities, memory loss, difficulty with problem solving and thinking, an increased heart rate, problems with *anxiety* (see Volume 2), and panic attacks. Long-term marijuana users may experience a physical dependence on marijuana, and WITHDRAWAL from the drug can cause anxiety, headaches, and nightmares.

Marijuana Users. In 1999 nearly 8 percent of American youths ages 12–17 reported using marijuana. Boys in that age range had a slightly higher rate of marijuana use (8.4 percent) than girls (7.1 percent). Use of the drug among youths is a source of concern. Researchers have found that adolescents who abuse marijuana are twice as likely as nonmarijuana users to skip school, steal items, attack others, and damage property.

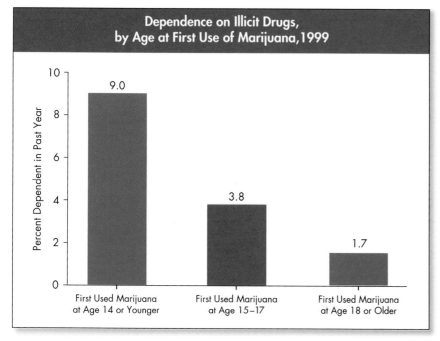

Dependence on Illicit Drugs, by Age at First Use of Marijuana, 1999

[Source: Substance Abuse and Mental Health Services Administration, *National Household Survey on Drug Abuse*, 1999.]

In recent years adolescents have become less concerned about the dangers of marijuana. Between 1996 and 1999, for example, the percentage of adolescents who said that smoking marijuana once a month was a great risk declined from about 33 percent to 29 percent. Experts are not certain why the perceptions of adolescents toward marijuana have changed, but the changing attitudes are a cause of worry.

While concern about the dangers of marijuana has declined among adolescents, emergency room visits related to marijuana abuse have risen dramatically, increasing from 15,706 visits in 1990 to 87,150 in 1999. Experts attribute this increase to the fact that most of the marijuana available today is much more potent than the varieties of the drug used in the past. According to the DRUG ENFORCEMENT ADMINISTRATION (DEA) the potency of marijuana today is up to 25 times greater than in past years.

Medicinal Uses of Marijuana. Some people advocate the use of marijuana for medicinal purposes, especially for people suffering from cancer, *AIDS* (see Volume 7), or the eye disease *glaucoma* (see Volume 8). Cancer and AIDS patients often suffer from extreme nausea, vomiting, and other side effects caused by the medications they take. Proponents of medicinal marijuana believe that marijuana can help relieve some of these side effects. In the case of glaucoma marijuana is thought to help relieve the eye pressure caused by this disease. In 1996 California passed a law allowing doctors to prescribe marijuana for medicinal purposes. However, the federal government does not acknowledge the validity of this law, and in 2001 the U.S. Supreme Court ruled that federal laws do not permit the use of marijuana for medicinal purposes.

There is some evidence that marijuana, rather than helping cancer sufferers, can be harmful to them. According to a study released in 2000 by the National Institute of Drug Abuse (NIDA), marijuana use can actually advance the growth of an existing cancerous tumor. In theory marijuana may also cause LUNG CANCER since the drug has higher concentrations of CARCINOGENS than TOBACCO. [*See also* DEPENDENCE, PHYSICAL; DRUG ABUSE; DRUGS AND HEALTH PROBLEMS.]

MEDICATIONS FOR ALCOHOL ADDICTION See ALCOHOL ADDICTION; ADDICTION, MEDICATIONS FOR.

MESCALINE An ILLEGAL DRUG derived from the juice of the peyote cactus. Mescaline is a HALLUCINOGEN, a mood-altering drug that can cause HALLUCINATIONS. The drug is generally taken orally or smoked, but on rare occasions it is injected. Mescaline is less potent than LSD, another well-known hallucinogen. Native Americans in northern Mexico and the southwestern United States sometimes use peyote in certain religious ceremonies.

METABOLISM OF ALCOHOL See ALCOHOL, METABOLISM OF.

METHADONE A synthetic NARCOTIC and a program to treat people addicted to HEROIN. Methadone has been used with heroin addicts since the 1970s. The drug suppresses the symptoms of heroin WITHDRAWAL and blocks the euphoric high that is produced by heroin.

Of the nearly 1 million heroin addicts in the United States, about 20 percent receive treatment with methadone. There are about 1,000 treatment programs throughout the nation—mostly in the larger cities—that can legally administer the drug. Some heroin addicts also get the drug illegally.

During the course of methadone treatment the drug is administered daily. LAAM (levomethadylacetate), a drug sometimes used in place of methadone, can be administered three times a week rather than daily. Researchers have discovered certain common factors among heroin addicts who are most likely to stay in methadone treatment. These include high motivation to avoid heroin, a court order requiring the individual to undergo treatment, no previous criminal record, psychological counseling, and an absence of other psychological problems.

Methadone has a number of advantages for drug abusers. Heroin addicts who use it are less likely to use heroin injected from dirty needles, thus reducing the risk of contracting HIV or HEPATITIS. They are also under the supervision of a doctor who can monitor their progress and overall health. A further advantage of methadone treatment is that, since methadone is a legal drug when obtained from a clinic, addicts are not forced to resort to crime to obtain the drug.

The major disadvantage of methadone treatment is that addicts who use the drug become dependent on it just as they do on heroin. Nevertheless, methadone is much less dangerous than heroin. Because of its addictive quality, many people remain on methadone for years. [*See also* ADDICTION; ADDICTION, MEDICATIONS FOR; ALCOHOL AND DRUG REHABILITATION PROGRAMS; DRUG ADDICTION.]

METHAMPHETAMINE Highly addictive synthetic STIMULANT that affects the central nervous system. Methamphetamine is an odorless, white crystalline powder that can be injected, inhaled (snorted), or swallowed. One form of the drug, called *ice*, is smoked.

Methamphetamine stimulates the release of brain chemicals called **dopamines**, which affect the pleasure center of the brain, causing a **rush**, or feeling of intense euphoria. Methamphetamine can continue to affect users for 6–8 hours after the drug is taken.

Keywords

dopamine chemical in the brain that helps transmit messages between brain cells
rush a sudden feeling of intense euphoria brought on by the use of certain drugs

If injected, the rush produced by the drug is almost instantaneous. When snorted, methamphetamine takes about 3–5 minutes to act. When consumed orally, the drug takes effect in about 15–20 minutes.

Short-term Effects. In addition to the typical rush produced by the drug, methamphetamine can also cause users to become agitated and to breathe heavily. Hyperactivity is another short-term effect. One of the most dangerous short-term effects of methamphetamine use is hyperthermia, an abnormally high body temperature that can be fatal if not treated by bringing down the temperature.

Long-term Effects. Regular methamphetamine abusers may become extremely agitated and violent. They are at increased risk for convulsions that can be fatal, and they often experience nausea, vomiting, insomnia, mental confusion, and memory loss. Long-term use of methamphetamine can create movement disorders that appear similar to ***Parkinson's disease*** (see Volume 8). Use of the drug may also cause HALLUCINATIONS, paranoia, and ***stroke*** (see Volume 8). Vital organs can be damaged by regular methamphetamine abuse. Damage to the heart can lead to HEART

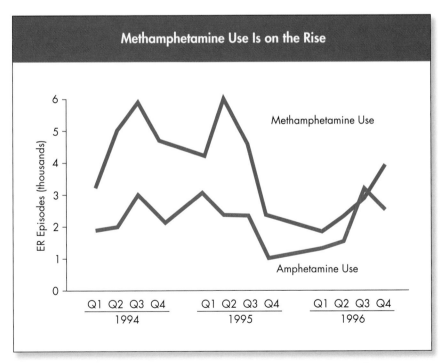

[Source: National Institute on Drug Abuse, *The Sixth Trienniel Report to Congress*, 1997.]

DISEASE, while damage to the brain can cause PSYCHOSIS that can last long after use of the drug has stopped. [See also DRUGS AND HEALTH PROBLEMS.]

MIXED DRINKS See ALCOHOL.

MORBIDITY AND MORTALITY, LEADING CAUSES OF See DEATH FROM ADDICTIONS.

NALTREXONE A prescribed medication approved by the Food and Drug Administration (FDA) in 1994 for treating ALCOHOL ADDICTION; also known as ReVia. Naltrexone was originally developed by the National Institute on Drug Abuse to treat HEROIN addicts, but it was later found to be effective with people addicted to ALCOHOL. Naltrexone blocks the pleasure centers of the brain from being stimulated by alcohol. As a result, people who take the drug and then drink will not have the pleasurable or euphoric feelings they may have felt in the past after consuming alcohol.

Studies have shown that alcoholics treated with naltrexone drink less often and are less likely to have a *relapse,* a return to using alcohol after attempting to give it up. The most effective use of naltrexone is to combine the drug with ABSTINENCE from all alcohol. Counseling for the alcoholic also enhances the success rate of the drug. [*See also* ALCOHOL ABUSE; ALCOHOL AND DRUG COUNSELING; ALCOHOL AND DRUG REHABILITATION PROGRAMS.]

NARCOTICS Drugs that act on the central nervous system, causing drowsiness and slowing down breathing. The word *narcotic* is derived from the Greek word for *stupor.* Most narcotics may be legally prescribed as painkilling medications for people suffering severe pain. One such drug is morphine, a drug derived from the juice of the opium poppy. However, some narcotics, such as HEROIN, are ILLEGAL DRUGS.

There are two main groups of narcotics: OPIATES such as opium, morphine, codeine, and heroin; and *opioids*—synthetic drugs such

Commonly Abused Drugs: Opioids

Substances	Examples of Proprietary or Street Names	Medical Uses	Route of Administration	DEA Schedules*	Period of Detection
CODEINE	TYLENOL W/CODEINE, ROBITUSSIN A-C, EMPIRIN W/CODEINE, FIORINAL W/CODEINE	ANALGESIC, ANTITUSSIVE	INJECTED, ORAL	II, III, IV	1–2 DAYS
HEROIN	DIACETYLMORPHINE; HORSE, SMACK	NONE	INJECTED, SMOKED, SNIFFED	I	1–2 DAYS
METHADONE	AMIDONE, DOLOPHINE, METHADOSE	ANALGESIC, TREATMENT FOR OPIATE DEPENDENCE	INJECTED, ORAL	II	1 DAY–1 WEEK
MORPHINE	ROXANOL, DURAMORPH	ANALGESIC	INJECTED, ORAL, SMOKED	II, III	1–2 DAYS
OPIUM	LAUDANUM, PAREGORIC; DOVER'S POWDER	ANALGESIC, ANTIDIARRHEAL	ORAL, SMOKED	II, III, V	1–2 DAYS

*Drug Enforcement Administration (DEA) Schedule I and II drugs have a high potential for abuse. They require greater storage security and have a quota on manufacture, among other restrictions. Schedule I drugs are available for research only and have no approved medical use. Schedule II drugs are available only through prescription, cannot have refills, and require a form for ordering. Schedule III and IV drugs are available with prescription, may have five refills in six months, and may be ordered verbally. Most Schedule V drugs are available over the counter.

[Source: National Institute on Drug Abuse, *Sixth Annual Report to Congress*, 2001.]

as METHADONE and Demerol, which are similar in their effect to the opiates. All narcotics have a high potential for causing ADDICTION, and as a result their use is highly controlled. The drugs are all listed as controlled substances by the DRUG ENFORCEMENT ADMINISTRATION (DEA). Heroin is the most commonly abused illegal narcotic in the United States.

When used in small, controlled doses, narcotics numb the senses, relieve severe pain and *anxiety* (see Volume 2), and induce sleep. They also produce a number of side effects, including constipation, nausea, and in some cases allergic reactions. When abused and taken in large doses, the drugs can be very dangerous, leading to stupor, convulsions, coma, and death.

Narcotics are often used appropriately and effectively as painkillers. In fact, studies show that hospital patients in severe pain who refuse to take narcotics recover more slowly from surgery than patients who take the drugs for pain relief. Competent physicians are well aware of the addiction potential of narcotics, and they carefully monitor use of the drugs and make sure to taper them off as soon as possible. Nevertheless, some patients do develop an addiction to narcotics. [*See also* DRUG ABUSE; DRUG ADDICTION.]

NICORETTE See NICOTINE REPLACEMENT THERAPY.

NICOTINE See TOBACCO, CHEMICALS IN.

NICOTINE REPLACEMENT THERAPY Methods for help with SMOKING CESSATION that use different products containing nicotine. There are several different forms of nicotine replacement therapy, all of which have been proven to be almost equally effective. In general, about 25–30 percent of smokers who have used nicotine replacement therapy are still not smoking a year later. This is about twice the rate of smokers who try to quit smoking with no medication or therapy.

Forms of Nicotine Replacement Therapy. The principle behind nicotine replacement therapy is that smokers will be able to stop smoking if the nicotine in the tobacco they use is replaced by nicotine found in a variety of nontobacco products.

One form of nicotine replacement therapy is the use of nicotine gum, such as Nicorette or other brands. These over-the-counter (OTC) products generally require about 1–2 months of use to help stop smoking.

Another nicotine replacement therapy uses the nicotine skin patch. Placed on the skin like a bandaid, the patch releases small amounts of nicotine that are absorbed into the skin and bloodstream. The patch may occasionally cause skin irritation. Nicotine patches are available as OTC drugs and are used for about 6 weeks. Some people use a combination of the nicotine skin patch and the antismoking drug Zyban. Studies indicate that this combination increases smoking cessation rates to 36–50 percent after one year.

Two other smoking cessation aids are the nicotine inhaler and nicotine nasal spray. Both of these are available only by prescription, and physicians determine the length of time that they should be used.

Personal Preferences and Choices. The effectiveness of the different forms of nicotine replacement therapy generally depends on personal preferences and choices. Some people dislike chewing nicotine gum because of its taste and prefer the patch, inhaler, or spray. Others find the gum easier to use than patches, inhalers, or sprays.

No matter what method an individual prefers and chooses, it is very important to follow the guidelines for each drug and avoid smoking while using them in order to avoid a buildup of nicotine in the body. This is particularly important for people with HEART DISEASE, since too much nicotine can raise blood pressure and cause the heart to work harder. [*See also* ADDICTION; ADDICTION, MEDICATIONS FOR.]

NONPRESCRIPTION DRUGS Medicinal drugs that can be purchased in pharmacies, supermarkets, convenience stores, and other locations; also known as over-the-counter (OTC) drugs. There are many different categories of OTC drugs, including antihistamines, laxatives, diet drugs, cough suppressants, analgesics, antidiarrhetics, and antacids. Many people assume that all nonprescription drugs are completely safe. However, it is possible to abuse these drugs just like ILLEGAL DRUGS.

Some individuals abuse over-the-counter cold and cough medicines, some of which contain substances that can create mild feelings of euphoria. If taken in large doses, abuse of these drugs can also result in seizures or panic attacks. Chronic use of high doses of such drugs can cause liver damage or brain damage. People abuse OTC drugs primarily by taking dosages above those recommended or by taking the drugs over long periods.

NUTRITION AND DRUG USE The effect of ILLEGAL DRUGS and ALCOHOL on food intake. People addicted to drugs or alcohol often have little or no interest in food. Instead, their primary concern is getting and using drugs or alcohol. Moreover, drug and alcohol abuse may impair the senses so that food does not smell or taste good, thus affecting a person's appetite. Because they have little interest in food, drug or alcohol abusers may become excessively thin. They also frequently develop various vitamin deficiencies and other health problems associated with poor nutrition, including *anemia* (see Volumes 4, 8), *scurvy* (see Volume 4), stomach disorders, and **malnutrition**. [*See also* ALCOHOL AND DRUGS, MALNUTRITION AND.]

OPIATES Drugs derived from the opium poppy, including opium, morphine, codeine, and HEROIN. Opiates act as DEPRESSANTS on the central nervous system, causing drowsiness and slowing down breathing. The potent drugs also numb the senses, which makes them powerful painkillers. If abused, opiates can cause stupor, convulsions, coma, and death.

Morphine and codeine are controlled but legal substances that are used primarily by physicians to control severe pain. However, other opiates, primarily heroin and opium, are used illegally by drug abusers seeking to attain a state of euphoria. Heroin is the most commonly abused opiate in the United States.

Because opiates have a high potential for abuse and ADDICTION, they are classified as **controlled substances** by the DRUG ENFORCEMENT ADMINISTRATION (DEA), which means that their legal availability and use are highly controlled and monitored. Most physicians are very careful about prescribing these drugs because of their potential for addiction. [*See also* DRUG ABUSE; DRUG ADDICTION; NARCOTICS.]

ORAL CANCER Cancer of the mouth or throat. About 30,000 new cases of oral cancer are diagnosed each year in the United States, and about 8,000 people die annually from the disease. An estimated 80 percent of oral cancers are attributed to smoking TOBACCO in cigarettes, cigars, or pipes, as well as to the use of SMOKELESS TOBACCO. Studies show that smokers who also drink excessive amounts of ALCOHOL may increase their risk of developing oral cancer.

The symptoms of oral cancer include a sore on the lip or inside the mouth that does not heal; unusual bleeding, pain, or numbness in the mouth; an abnormal change in the voice; a sore throat that does not go away; and difficulty or pain in swallowing or chewing. If treated early, oral cancer can often be cured. Standard treatment involves removing cancer tumors surgically or treating them with radiation to kill cancerous growths. [*See also* THROAT CANCER; TOBACCO AND HEALTH PROBLEMS.]

OVERDOSE See ALCOHOL OVERDOSE; DRUG OVERDOSE.

P

PCP An ILLEGAL DRUG that is a HALLUCINOGEN; also commonly known as angel dust. PCP (phencyclidine) was originally developed in the 1950s as an anesthetic drug for humans. In the 1960s it was also used as a sedating drug for animals. Taken off the market in 1965 because of potentially harmful side effects, PCP is now illegal.

PCP is one of many PSYCHOACTIVE DRUGS. Found as either a powder or a liquid, the drug may cause users to feel detached and numbed as well as extremely strong and invulnerable. PCP users may experience visual and auditory HALLUCINATIONS, severe mood disorders, and **amnesia**. The drug can also cause paranoia and hostility as well as PSYCHOSIS in some users. The psychotic symptoms associated with PCP are sometimes very similar to *schizophrenia* (see Volume 2), a severe mental disorder.

Keywords

amnesia a complete or partial loss of memory
hernia a protrusion of an organ or tissue through an opening in its surrounding walls, especially in the abdominal region of the body
psychoactive capable of causing dramatic mood changes

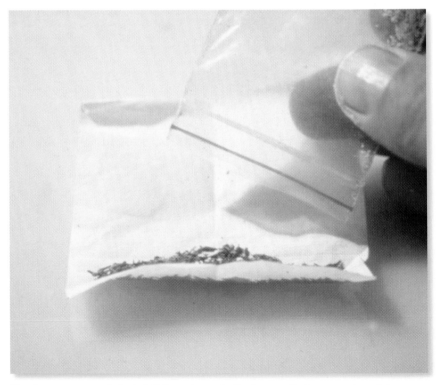

Also known as angel dust, PCP is a strong hallucinogen that can produce intense hostility in some users.

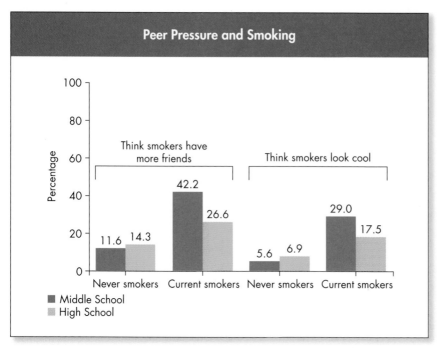

Peer Pressure and Smoking

Think smokers have more friends

Think smokers look cool

- Never smokers: 11.6 (Middle School), 14.3 (High School)
- Current smokers: 42.2 (Middle School), 26.6 (High School)
- Never smokers: 5.6 (Middle School), 6.9 (High School)
- Current smokers: 29.0 (Middle School), 17.5 (High School)

Middle School
High School

[Source: U.S. Department of Health and Human Services, *Youth Tobacco Surveillance United States, 1998–1999,* 2000.]

PEER PRESSURE AND ADDICTION Pressure from friends or other individuals of about the same age to use ALCOHOL, TOBACCO, or ILLEGAL DRUGS. According to the Office of the Surgeon General, acceptance by their peers is very important to adolescents ages 11 to 15. Adolescents who drink, smoke, or take drugs may encourage, taunt, or dare other teens to try these activities as well. Younger adolescents may also look upon older peers or siblings as role models and attempt to copy their behaviors, including the use of addicting substances.

Adolescents are more likely to smoke, drink, or take drugs if they believe that these activities are a way of becoming or remaining an accepted member of a group that is important to them, or if the activities make them feel more adult. Smoking, drinking, or taking drugs becomes a rite of passage, an act showing that an adolescent is no longer a child.

Although it can be difficult, teens can develop stategies to resist peer pressure. Responding to taunts or dares in a joking way can sometimes be effective. But if the pressure to conform continues, just firmly saying "no" can be very effective.

POISONING, DRUG AND ALCOHOL OVERDOSE See ALCOHOL POISONING; ALCOHOL OVERDOSE; DRUG OVERDOSE; Volume 2.

PREGNANCY AND TOBACCO, ALCOHOL, AND DRUGS The effects of addicting substances on the mother and fetus during **pregnancy** (see Volume 3). The use of TOBACCO, ALCOHOL, or DRUGS during pregnancy can be very harmful to an expectant mother and her developing fetus. As a result, pregnant

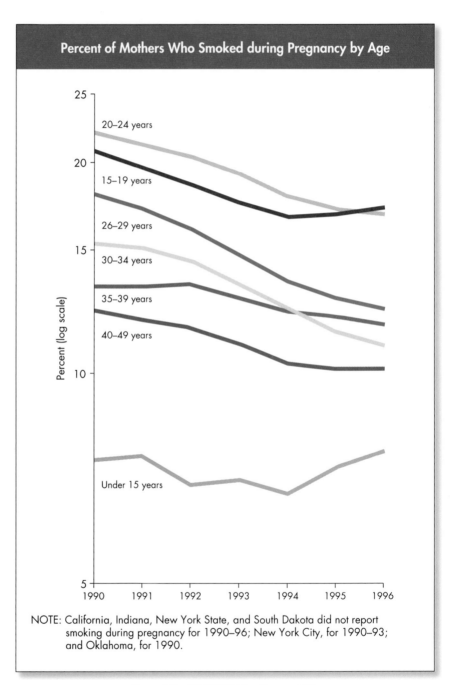

Percent of Mothers Who Smoked during Pregnancy by Age

NOTE: California, Indiana, New York State, and South Dakota did not report smoking during pregnancy for 1990–96; New York City, for 1990–93; and Oklahoma, for 1990.

[Source: *National Vital Statistics Reports*, 47, 10, 1998.]

women should not smoke, consume alcohol, or use any drugs other than those prescribed by a medical doctor at any time during pregnancy. Exposure of the fetus to these substances can result in various birth defects or can cause an infant to be stillborn, or born dead.

Effects of Alcohol. Regular or heavy consumption of alcohol during pregnancy can cause FETAL ALCOHOL SYNDROME (FAS), which can result in mental retardation, *cerebral palsy* (see Volume 8), heart defects, kidney problems, and hernias. Learning delays are also common among children with FAS.

Effects of Drugs. Many drugs, both legal and illegal, have the potential to harm a fetus, especially in the first trimester (first three months of pregnancy), when the brain and nervous system are developing. ILLEGAL DRUGS can cause a number of serious problems in a developing fetus. For example, the use of MARIJUANA or HASHISH during pregnancy can cause birth defects. Infants born to mothers who abuse AMPHETAMINES may suffer from damage to their central nervous system. OPIATES such as HEROIN can cause fetal death or death to a newborn born prematurely. Many babies born to drug-abusing mothers are of low birthweight and slow to develop. When born addicted to drugs, infants must undergo the tremendous strain of drug WITHDRAWAL after enduring the trauma of childbirth.

Effects of Tobacco. Exposure to tobacco is also very dangerous for a developing fetus. The nicotine ingested by a smoking mother crosses immediately through the placenta and is absorbed by the fetus. The carbon monoxide in tobacco smoke can interfere with the oxygen supply to the fetus, causing serious brain damage.

Pregnant women who smoke also risk premature deliveries and low-birthweight babies. Some evidence suggests that maternal tobacco use may cause some birth defects, and smoking is also linked to an increased risk for sudden infant death syndrome (SIDS), a tragic circumstance in which a newborn baby suddenly dies for no apparent reason. [*See also* ALCOHOL AND HEALTH PROBLEMS; DRUGS AND HEALTH PROBLEMS; TOBACCO AND HEALTH PROBLEMS.]

PSYCHOACTIVE DRUGS Legal or ILLEGAL DRUGS that can alter a person's moods or behavior. Virtually all addictive drugs are psychoactive—that is, they are capable of causing dramatic mood changes. Often the very reason a person becomes addicted to a drug is because of the psychoactive effects it causes. Many drugs, including various STIMULANTS, induce a state of euphoria, or a high. Others, such as DEPRESSANTS, take away a person's normal inhibitions and fears.

Legally prescribed medications may also be abused for their psychoactive effects. Antidepressants prescribed for people with *depression* (see Volume 2) or antipsychotic medicines given to people with *mental illness* (see Volume 2) are examples of legal psychoactive drugs. NARCOTICS, which include legal substances like morphine and codeine, as well as illegal drugs such as HEROIN, are also psychoactive drugs.

Most HALLUCINOGENS are psychoactive, giving users a false sense of power or a feeling of euphoria. AMPHETAMINES provide a stimulating psychoactive effect as well as a euphoric high, while INHALANTS, which are abused primarily by teenagers, may cause an elevated mood. Use of any psychoactive drug carries various health risks, particularly the use of illegal drugs or the abuse of certain prescribed drugs. [*See also* DRUGS AND HEALTH PROBLEMS.]

PSYCHOSIS Severe temporary or long-term *mental illness* (see Volume 2) affecting the total personality, in which individuals lose contact with reality and may pose a threat to themselves or to others. People suffering from psychosis may have delusions of persecution or think that they can fly off high buildings or perform other miraculous feats. They may also be extremely fearful or exhibit violent rages. Some drugs, including HALLUCINOGENS, ANABOLIC STEROIDS, and METHAMPHETAMINE, may induce either temporary or more long-term psychosis. Individuals going through WITHDRAWAL from ALCOHOL and suffering from DELIRIUM TREMENS (DTs) may also experience psychosis. [*See also* DRUGS AND HEALTH PROBLEMS.]

RAVES Large parties attended primarily by adolescents and young adults that involve very loud music and much dancing, usually combined with the abuse of ALCOHOL and DRUGS. DESIGNER DRUGS or CLUB DRUGS are very popular at raves, as are other ILLEGAL DRUGS such as MARIJUANA, PCP, LSD, and COCAINE.

Raves can be very risky social gatherings because of the easy availability of drugs and the uninhibited atmosphere that is typical of these parties. Some people at raves take many different drugs, sometimes several at a time, not knowing what any of the drugs are or their dosages. The quality of the illegal drugs at the parties is generally unknown, and sometimes they may contain toxic or poisonous chemicals. The potential for DRUG OVERDOSE is high at raves, and the combination of alcohol and drugs as well as the potential risks of harmful DRUG INTERACTIONS only increase the danger.

Raves pose another danger as well. Because drugs are often passed around freely, individuals are at risk of unknowingly being given DATE RAPE DRUGS amidst the chaos and confusion. Taking these drugs will put them at increased risk of *sexual assault* or *rape* (see Volume 5). [*See also* ALCOHOL, DRUG/MEDICATION INTER-ACTIONS WITH.]

S

SECONDHAND SMOKE Smoke produced by a smoker that is harmful to others; sometimes known also as environmental tobacco smoke. Secondhand smoke includes **side-stream smoke**, which a smoker blows into the air and nonsmokers inhale. It also includes the smoke that comes from any lit cigarette, cigar, or pipe that is left unattended or is just being held by a smoker. Those who breathe in secondhand smoke are said to experience **passive smoking**.

Secondhand smoke poses a health risk to anyone who inhales it. According to the *Environmental Protection Agency (EPA)* (see Volume 6), exposure to secondhand smoke can cause LUNG CANCER. Experts estimate that environmental tobacco smoke causes about 3,000 lung cancer deaths each year among nonsmokers.

Secondhand smoke has also been linked to HEART DISEASE as well as to ASTHMA and respiratory problems in children. According to the U.S. Surgeon General, each year in the United States children get at least 150,000 respiratory infections such as BRONCHITIS and *pneumonia* (see Volume 8) as a result of breathing in secondhand smoke. [*See also* SURGEON GENERAL'S WARNINGS; TOBACCO AND HEALTH PROBLEMS; TOBACCO AND RESPIRATORY DISEASES.]

Keywords

antibodies substances made by the body to attack foreign organisms or chemicals
passive smoking breathing in secondhand smoke, or smoke that is generated by another person
side-stream smoke the smoke that a nonsmoker inhales from the environment

Summary of Landmark Events in the Development of U.S. Policies for Clean Indoor Air

Year	Event
1971	The Surgeon General proposes a federal smoking ban in public places.
1972	The first report of the Surgeon General to identify environmental tobacco smoke (ETS) as a health risk is released.
1973	Arizona becomes the first state to restrict smoking in several public places and to reduce ETS exposure because it is a health risk.
	The Civil Aeronautics Board requires no-smoking sections on all commercial airline flights.
1974	Connecticut passes the first state law to apply smoking restrictions to restaurants.
1975	Minnesota passes a comprehensive statewide law for clean indoor air.
1977	Berkeley, California, becomes the first community to limit smoking in restaurants and other public places.
1983	San Francisco passes a law to place private workplaces under smoking restrictions.
1986	A report of the Surgeon General focuses entirely on the health consequences of involuntary smoking; ETS is proclaimed a cause of lung cancer in healthy nonsmokers.
	The National Academy of Sciences issues a report on the health consequences of involuntary smoking.
	Americans for Nonsmokers' Rights becomes a national group; it had originally formed as California GASP (Group to Alleviate Smoking Pollution).
1987	The U.S. Department of Health and Human Services establishes a smoke-free environment in all of its buildings, affecting 120,000 employees nationwide.
	Minnesota passes a law requiring all hospitals in the state to ban smoking by 1990.
	A Gallup poll finds, for the first time, that a majority (55 percent) of all U.S. adults favor a complete ban on smoking in all public places.
1988	A congressionally mandated smoking ban takes effect on all domestic airline flights of two hours or less.
	New York City's ordinance for clean indoor air takes effect, banning or severely limiting smoking in various public places and affecting 7 million people.
	California implements a statewide ban on smoking aboard all intrastate airplane, train, and bus trips.
1990	A congressionally mandated smoking ban takes effect on all domestic airline flights of six hours or less.
	The U.S. Environmental Protection Agency (EPA) issues a draft risk-assessment on ETS.
1991	CDC's National Institute for Occupational Safety and Health issues a bulletin recommending that secondhand smoke be reduced to the lowest feasible concentration in the workplace.
1992	Hospitals applying for accreditation by the Joint Commission on the Accreditation of Healthcare Organizations are required to develop a policy to prohibit smoking by patients, visitors, employees, volunteers, and medical staff.
	The EPA releases its report classifying ETS as a group A (known human) carcinogen, placing ETS in the same category as asbestos, benzene, and radon.

Summary of Landmark Events in the Development of U.S. Policies for Clean Indoor Air

1993	LOS ANGELES PASSES A BAN ON SMOKING IN ALL RESTAURANTS.
	THE U.S. POSTAL SERVICE ELIMINATES SMOKING IN ALL FACILITIES.
	CONGRESS ENACTS A SMOKE-FREE POLICY FOR WIC (SPECIAL SUPPLEMENTAL FOOD PROGRAM FOR WOMEN, INFANTS, AND CHILDREN) CLINICS.
	A WORKING GROUP OF 16 STATE ATTORNEYS GENERAL RELEASES RECOMMENDATIONS FOR ESTABLISHING SMOKE-FREE POLICIES IN FAST-FOOD RESTAURANTS.
	VERMONT BANS SMOKING IN ALL PUBLIC BUILDINGS AND MANY PRIVATE BUILDINGS OPEN TO THE PUBLIC.
1994	THE U.S. DEPARTMENT OF DEFENSE PROHIBITS SMOKING IN ALL INDOOR MILITARY FACILITIES.
	THE OCCUPATIONAL SAFETY AND HEALTH ADMINISTRATION PROPOSES A RULE THAT WOULD BAN SMOKING IN MOST U.S. WORKPLACES.
	SAN FRANCISCO PASSES A BAN ON SMOKING IN ALL RESTAURANTS AND WORKPLACES.
	THE PRO-CHILDREN'S ACT REQUIRES PERSONS PROVIDING FEDERALLY FUNDED CHILDREN'S SERVICES TO PROHIBIT SMOKING IN THOSE FACILITIES.
1995	NEW YORK CITY PASSES A COMPREHENSIVE ORDINANCE EFFECTIVELY BANNING SMOKING IN MOST WORKPLACES.
	MARYLAND ENACTS A SMOKE-FREE POLICY FOR ALL WORKPLACES EXCEPT HOTELS, BARS, RESTAURANTS, AND PRIVATE CLUBS.
	CALIFORNIA PASSES COMPREHENSIVE LEGISLATION THAT PROHIBITS SMOKING IN MOST ENCLOSED WORKPLACES.
	VERMONT'S SMOKING BAN IS EXTENDED TO INCLUDE RESTAURANTS, BARS, HOTELS, AND MOTELS, EXCEPT THOSE HOLDING A CABARET LICENSE.
1996	THE U.S. DEPARTMENT OF TRANSPORTATION REPORTS THAT ABOUT 80 PERCENT OF NONSTOP SCHEDULED U.S. AIRLINE FLIGHTS BETWEEN THE UNITED STATES AND FOREIGN POINTS WILL BE SMOKE-FREE BY JUNE 1, 1996.
1997	PRESIDENT CLINTON SIGNS AN EXECUTIVE ORDER ESTABLISHING A SMOKE-FREE ENVIRONMENT FOR FEDERAL EMPLOYEES AND ALL MEMBERS OF THE PUBLIC VISITING FEDERALLY OWNED FACILITIES.
	THE CALIFORNIA EPA ISSUES A REPORT DETERMINING THAT ETS IS A TOXIC AIR CONTAMINANT.
	SETTLEMENT IS REACHED IN THE CLASS-ACTION LAWSUIT BROUGHT BY FLIGHT ATTENDANTS EXPOSED TO ETS.
1998	THE U.S. SENATE BANS SMOKING IN THE SENATE'S PUBLIC SPACES.
	CALIFORNIA LAW TAKES EFFECT BANNING SMOKING IN BARS UNLESS A BAR HAS A SEPARATELY VENTILATED SMOKING AREA.

[Source: Centers for Disease Control and Prevention, *Reducing Tobacco Use: A Report of the Surgeon General*, 2000.]

SIDE-STREAM SMOKE See SECONDHAND SMOKE.

SMOKELESS TOBACCO TOBACCO products that are not smoked, such as chewing tobacco or snuff. Chewing tobacco consists of roughly cut tobacco leaves that are held between the cheek and gum. This "wad" or "chaw" of tobacco is sucked and chewed. Snuff, a finely ground, moist form of tobacco, is usually placed between the lower lip and gum, where it mixes with saliva.

Smokeless tobacco is popular among some adolescents and young adults. For example, among students in American middle schools about 3.5 percent of males and 1.4 percent of females have used some form of smokeless tobacco. The use of smokeless tobacco differs somewhat by race or ethnic group. Among high school students, for example, about 10 percent of white students use smokeless tobacco, compared to about 4 percent of Hispanic students and 1 percent of African American students.

Some smokeless tobacco products are flavored with cherry or apple juice, honey, or even chocolate liqueur by tobacco companies, which makes them more appealing to new users. These flavored forms of smokeless tobacco are also often lower in nicotine and appeal more to new users who do not like the harsh taste of tobacco products with heavier concentrations of nicotine. When users of smokeless tobacco become addicted as well as accustomed to the taste and effect of tobacco, many of them move on to brands with higher levels of nicotine.

The use of smokeless tobacco carries a number of health risks. In addition to causing gum disease, these products also increase the risk of ORAL CANCER, cancer of the esophagus, and HEART DISEASE. [*See also* TOBACCO AND HEALTH PROBLEMS; TOBACCO, CHEMICALS IN.]

SMOKING CESSATION Ending the use of TOBACCO in any form—cigarettes, cigars, pipes, or SMOKELESS TOBACCO. Most people who smoke or use smokeless tobacco eventually decide that they want to quit, usually for health reasons. Once a person is addicted to nicotine, however, it is not easy to stop using tobacco—but it is possible.

Studies have shown that most smokers need some help in order to stop using tobacco, either with NICOTINE REPLACEMENT THERAPY, medications such as Zyban, or some other form of therapy. About a million smokers in the United States stop smoking each year, but 75 percent of them relapse, or return to using tobacco after attempting to give it up. When a smoking cessation aid such as nicotine replacement therapy or medications is added, the success rate is doubled, according to the Office of the Surgeon General.

Nicotine Replacement Therapy. Some people succeed in ending their tobacco habit with nicotine replacement therapy, a method that delivers nicotine to the body through the use of nicotine gum, skin patches, nasal sprays, or inhalers. These nicotine replacement devices are about equally effective; about 30 percent of those who use this therapy remain off tobacco. Each method has a few drawbacks. Nicotine gum may cause some minor indigestion, and some people dislike the taste. The skin patch has been know to cause minor skin irritation. The nasal spray produces the most side effects, causing runny noses, sneezing, watery eyes, and coughing.

Zyban. Zyban, also known as bupropion, is an effective medication for many people wishing to stop smoking. This drug is also used as an antidepressant, although smokers who wish to quit need not be depressed to succeed with the medication. Zyban should not be taken by people who have a history of seizures because it could make the seizures worse. The main side effects with this drug are dry mouth and insomnia. Studies have shown that about 30 percent of those who took Zyban were still off tobacco a year later. If ex-smokers use a combination of Zyban and nicotine skin patches, the success rate increases to about 36 percent.

Rapid Smoking. One form of smoking cessation treatment is to have the smoker inhale very deeply and smoke very quickly to the point of nausea. This method is known as "rapid smoking." A physician supervises this treatment in case the person becomes very ill. The treatment generally is not used with older people or those with heart problems because it can put a strain on the lungs and heart. Studies by the Office of the Surgeon General have found that rapid smoking succeeded in about 40 percent of those who tried the method; those 40 percent were still not smoking 6–12 months after treatment ended. Not many physicians are willing to provide this treatment, however, because of its effect on the heart and lungs.

Alternative Methods of Smoking Cessation. Hypnotherapy is another treatment to help smokers quit using tobacco. In this method the individual is placed in a light trance by a trained hypnotherapist, who offers hypnotic suggestions guiding the person to avoid tobacco. Although some people seem to respond to hypnotherapy, there is not yet enough evidence to determine whether or not this method is effective.

Acupuncture is another method that some smokers have tried in order to end their tobacco habit. This type of therapy involves the mostly painless insertion of very thin needles at certain points on the body. The needles are thought to stimulate or repress the central nervous system in various ways. For the most part, studies have not shown acupuncture to be effective. However, this alternative therapy is gaining in popularity for the treatment of various other ailments.

Scientists are currently studying immunization therapy as a possible treatment for people addicted to tobacco. This method of therapy would involve injecting a vaccine that could create **antibodies** to prevent nicotine from reaching the brain, thus reducing the desire for the drug. Immunization research on animals using a nicotine-blocking vaccine has been promising. If the therapy proves effective for humans, it will be easier to quit smoking because people will be able get a series of injections to eliminate their addiction. [*See also* TOBACCO ADDICTION.]

SPIT TOBACCO See SMOKELESS TOBACCO.

STIMULANTS Drugs that stimulate the central nervous system, causing increased activity in the muscles and nerves. Stimulants

Commonly Abused Drugs: Stimulants

Substances	Examples of Proprietary or Street Names	Medical Uses	Route of Administration	DEA Schedules*	Period of Detection
AMPHETAMINE	BIPHETAMINE, DEXEDRINE; BLACK BEAUTIES, CROSSES, HEARTS	ATTENTION DEFICIT HYPERACTIVITY DISORDER (ADHD), OBESITY, NARCOLEPSY	INJECTED, ORAL, SMOKED, SNIFFED	II	1–2 DAYS
COCAINE	COKE, CRACK, FLAKE, ROCKS, SNOW	LOCAL ANESTHETIC, VASOCONSTRICTOR	INJECTED, SMOKED, SNIFFED	II	1–4 DAYS
METHAMPHETAMINE	DESOXYN; CRANK, CRYSTAL, GLASS, ICE, SPEED	ADHD, OBESITY, NARCOLEPSY	INJECTED, ORAL, SMOKED, SNIFFED	II	1–2 DAYS
METHYLPHENIDATE	RITALIN	ADHD, NARCOLEPSY	INJECTED, ORAL	II	1–2 DAYS
NICOTINE	HABITROL PATCH, NICORETTE GUM, NICOTROL SPRAY, PROSTEP PATCH, CIGARS, CIGARETTES, SMOKELESS TOBACCO, SNUFF, SPIT TOBACCO	TREATMENT FOR NICOTINE DEPENDENCE	SMOKED, SNIFFED, ORAL, TRANSDERMAL	NOT SCHEDULED	1–2 DAYS

[Source: National Institute on Drug Abuse, *Sixth Annual Report to Congress*, 2001.]

increase alertness and speed up the heart rate. They induce a temporary feeling of well-being as well as provide relief from fatigue. Two of the most common stimulants, used daily by millions of people, are caffeine (found in coffee, tea, and various soft drinks) and nicotine (found in tobacco). In addition to these legal substances there are various ILLEGAL DRUGS that are stimulants, including COCAINE, CRACK COCAINE, AMPHETAMINES, and METHAMPHETAMINE.

Abuse of stimulants can lead to ADDICTION, and the drugs pose a number of health risks. Heavy use of caffeine, for example, can cause headaches, irritability, tremors, and nervousness, while very large amounts can even cause HALLUCINATIONS and perhaps convulsions. In addition to being highly addictive, nicotine can damage the cardiovascular system, which includes the heart and blood vessels. Illegal stimulants are even more dangerous, posing health threats at much lower doses than caffeine or nicotine. Among the dangers of these illegal drugs are heart attacks, heart *arrythmia* (see Volume 8), seizures, PSYCHOSIS, hallucinations, paranoia, violent behavior, and even death. [*See also* DRUGS AND HEALTH PROBLEMS; TOBACCO AND HEALTH PROBLEMS; TOBACCO AND RESPIRATORY PROBLEMS.]

SUBSTANCE ABUSE See ALCOHOL ABUSE; DRUG ABUSE.

SUPPORT GROUPS Organizations that provide support for people with particular problems. There are support groups for people dealing with virtually any type of problem, including addictions such as alcoholism and other types of substance abuse.

Types of Support Groups. Some support groups are advocacy groups, mainly providing information about problems and how to get help for them. Other support groups are self-help groups, in which people with a particular problem meet regularly and give each other encouragement and advice. Some support groups are both advocacy and self-help groups. Most support groups have national toll-free numbers, Web sites, and e-mail addresses to contact for assistance.

Advocacy Groups. Advocacy groups provide detailed, up-to-date information about a problem, such as its causes, risk factors, and rates or occurrence. They also usually have information on treatment resources across the country and the latest treatment options. In addition, many advocacy goups work to heighten public awareness of the problem and to fight for the rights of people with the problem. Examples of advocacy groups are the National

Eating Disorders Organization, National Foundation for Depressive Illness, National Alliance for the Mentally Ill, and Anxiety Disorders Association of America.

Self-Help Groups Self-help groups provide members with acceptance, moral support, and practical advice on coping with their mutual problem. For many people simply sharing their concerns and experiences with others who have the same problem is extremely helpful. Many national self-help groups have local meetings all over the country. The best known self-help group is ALCOHOLICS ANONYMOUS (AA). Others include Narcotics Anonymous, Gamblers Anonymous, and Obsessive-Compulsive Anonymous.

Alcoholics Anonymous was the first successful self-help group, and many other self-help groups are modeled on it. AA's TWELVE-STEP PROGRAM has been adopted by many other self-help groups, including Gamblers Anonymous and Obsessive-Compulsive Anonymous. It is based on the personal experiences of AA's founding members and serves as a guide to new members as they struggle to abstain from alcohol for life. [*See also* AL-ANON; ALA-TEEN; ALCOHOL AND MENTAL HEALTH; SOCIAL SUPPORT SYSTEMS.]

MORE SOURCES See www. alcoholics-anonymous.org; www.psych central.com

SURGEON GENERAL'S WARNINGS Alerts issued by the Office of the Surgeon General of the United States advising American of the dangers of TOBACCO. As early as 1956 the Office of the Surgeon General reported on the link between excessive smoking and LUNG CANCER. In 1964 the Surgeon General released the *First Report on Smoking and Health*, which reported that smoking caused lung cancer. Today, each package of cigarettes contains a warning from the Surgeon General about the dangers of smoking.

In 1994 the Surgeon General identified a number of risk factors that lead adolescents to use tobacco—the perception that tobacco use is normal, use of tobacco by friends and siblings, and the belief that tobacco provides benefits. The Surgeon General also reported that, in terms of SMOKELESS TOBACCO, teenagers continue to use this type of product because of a lack of knowledge about its harmful effects. Concerned over continued use of tobacco among teens, the federal government established regulations in 1996 that banned the sale of tobacco to anyone under the age of 18. [*See also* TOBACCO AND HEALTH PROBLEMS; TOBACCO AND RESPIRATORY DISEASES; TOBACCO LAWS.]

T

TAR See TOBACCO, CHEMICALS IN.

TEENS AND ADDICTION The psychological and physical dependence of adolescents on ALCOHOL, DRUGS, or TOBACCO. In many cases adolescents who abuse one substance will also abuse others. For example, teenagers who smoke are much more likely to drink alcohol or to use ILLEGAL DRUGS than are nonsmokers.

Teens and Alcohol Abuse. Although most adolescents between the ages of 12 and 17 do not drink, about a third of teenagers do, often quite regularly. Drinking begins for these young people at age 14 or 15, and about 40 percent of drinking adolescents will become addicted to alcohol.

Risk Factors. According to the National Institute on Alcohol Abuse and Alcoholism, a number of factors play a significant role in adolescents developing ALCOHOL ADDICTION. Among the most important of these factors is home life. Parents who are heavy drinkers or alcoholics or who pay little attention to their children's activities may foster teen drinking. Additionally, parental rejection, childhood abuse, or other trauma can lead to adolescent alcohol abuse.

Young people who begin using alcohol or drugs before age 15 are also at high risk for alcohol abuse, as are those whose friends use alcohol or drugs. Other risk factors for adolescents are aggressive and antisocial behavior and poor performance in school. The more of these factors present in an adolescent's life, the greater the risk of addiction to alcohol.

Risky Behavior. Adolescent alcohol abusers often report that they have acted in ways that they later regretted and that alcohol made it difficult for them to think clearly. Drinking teens, for instance, often have poor school attendance and grades. They frequently engage in early *sexual activity* as well as in *unprotected sex* (see Volume 7). They also become victims of violent crimes, such as *assault, rape* (see Volume 5), and robbery.

Some 8 percent of teen drinkers engage in another risky practice, BINGE DRINKING, or very heavy drinking within a certain period of time. Binge drinking is very dangerous because it can lead to ALCOHOL POISONING, which can be fatal.

Teens Who Abuse Alcohol. Adolescent males are heavier alcohol abusers than females. For example, in a study of high school seniors, 39 percent of the boys said they had been drunk in the past 30 days versus 29 percent of the girls.

When considering ethnic background and heavy drinking, white teens lead other adolescent heavy drinkers, followed by Hispanics. Fewer than 1 percent of black teenagers are heavy drinkers.

Teens and Drug Addiction. Most adolescents are not addicted to drugs, nor do they abuse them. However, some 11 percent of those aged 12–17 used illegal drugs in 1999. In a nationwide study of high school students and addictive behaviors researchers found that 4 percent of the students had used COCAINE one or more times in the month prior to the survey. About 5 percent of the males and 3 percent of the females reported current cocaine use. Hispanic and white students (at 7 percent and 4 percent, respectively) were most likely to be cocaine abusers. Only about 1 percent of African Americans students had used cocaine in the period covered by the study.

The study also showed that about 15 percent of the students had used INHALANTS. White and Hispanic students, at about 16 percent each, were much more likely than black students, at about 5 percent, to use these drugs.

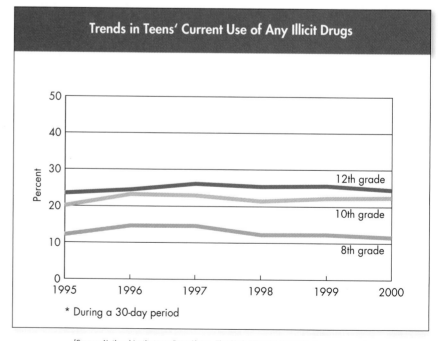

[Source: National Institute on Drug Abuse, *The Sixth Triennial Report to Congress*, 1997.]

When researchers asked about the abuse of other drugs, they discovered that 9 percent of the students had used METHAMPHET-AMINE. The main users of this drug were Hispanics (11 percent) and whites (10 percent), while only 2 percent of black students admitted to taking the drug.

Teens and Tobacco. The average age that adolescents start using tobacco is 12 years old. The majority of adults who smoke report that they too began smoking in their early teens.

In general, most smoking-related health problems, such as LUNG CANCER, HEART DISEASE, and EMPHYSEMA, do not plague young smokers. However, teenage girls who smoke may experience painful menstrual periods. In the future those who continue to smoke will face the various health consequences associated with smoking.

Despite these risks, teen female smokers may not wish to quit because they fear gaining weight. Studies indicate that weight gains of up to 10 pounds can occur. However, active exercise combined with NICOTINE REPLACEMENT THERAPY or with taking Zyban can limit this weight gain.

White adolescents are the heaviest users of tobacco, with about 27 percent smoking cigarettes. They are followed by Hispanics at about 20 percent and then African American teens, at about 16 percent. Of white adolescent tobacco users some 28 percent report also smoking cigars, compared to 16 percent of black teens.

When it comes to SMOKELESS TOBACCO, about 8 percent of teens have either used chewing tobacco or snuff. Around 10 percent of white students use smokeless tobacco, compared to about 4 percent of Hispanic and 1 percent of African American students. Males are much more likely (by about 14 to 1) to use smokeless tobacco products than females.

Why Teens Abuse Substances. Experts who have studied why adolescents begin using addictive substances have discovered a number of factors. One important reason for abuse is the desire for social approval, and often adolescents encourage friends to try a can of beer, a cigarette, or perhaps some marijuana or cocaine. Researchers have found that teaching teenagers how to say no to their friends can be an effective way to limit abuse of alcohol, drugs, or tobacco.

Sensation-seeking is another reason for abuse. Teenagers may want excitement or novelty and may believe that forbidden substances such as drugs, alcohol, or tobacco will provide the sensations they desire. If the experience is sufficiently exciting, a teenager will try again, and addiction often follows.

Adolescent Drinking Compared to Percentage Using Illegal Drugs and Smoking				
	Nondrinkers	**Drinkers**	**Bingers**	**Heavy Drinkers**
ILLEGAL DRUG USE	3.3	25.6	43.2	52.7
SMOKING	10.5	44.1	63.6	76.0

[Source: Janet C. Greenblatt, "Patterns of Alcohol Use Among Adolescents and Associations with Emotional and Behavioral Problems," 2000.]

Some teens have role models in their families who abuse drugs, alcohol, and tobacco. Thus, the adolescent may see this behavior as normal and acceptable. Emotional or *mental illness* (see Volume 2) may also lead to addiction. The depressed or anxious teenager may be seeking something, anything, to relieve internal *stress* or *anxiety* (see Volume 2).

Treating Addicted Teens. It is very hard to break the cycle of substance abuse unless the individual wishes to do so. Adolescents may not have the maturity to understand this; and when they are abusing drugs or alcohol, their judgment is also impaired. However, parents or legal guardians may be able to coerce teens to undergo treatment, an option not usually available to the families of adults who abuse drugs or alcohol. A TWELVE-STEP PROGRAM may also be effective, especially if the teenager is a regular attendee at meetings.

With tobacco, successful treatment for teenage addictions may include the use of ANTISMOKING PRODUCTS, such as nicotine gum, a nasal spray or inhaler, or a skin patch. HYPNOTHERAPY may also be a reasonable option if the teenager is willing to try it. Likewise, group or individual therapy may help. Some antismoking clinics have had success with alternative remedies, such as acupuncture. A further aid is if family members who smoke end their own smoking habits.

THROAT CANCER Cancer of the larynx, or voicebox. About 12,000 Americans are diagnosed with throat cancer each year. The disease is most common among smokers, particularly those who are also abusers of ALCOHOL. Throat cancer is about four times more common among men than women and is found more frequently among African American males. [*See also* TOBACCO AND HEALTH PROBLEMS; TOBACCO AND RESPIRATORY DISEASES.]

TOBACCO A plant whose leaves are processed to make tobacco products, primarily for smoking. Tobacco is one of the most abused substances in the world. In the United States alone more than 66 million people used one or more forms of tobacco in 1999. Of these, 57 million smoked cigarettes, about 12 million smoked cigars, 7.6 million used some form of SMOKELESS TOBACCO, and about 2.4 million used pipe tobacco.

Tobacco is responsible for about 430,000 deaths each year in the United States, and the medical costs related to smoking are at least $50 billion annually. Tobacco use has been shown to increase the risk of certain types of cancers, including LUNG CANCER and THROAT CANCER. Smoking and SECONDHAND SMOKE also cause or worsen such diseases as ASTHMA and BRONCHITIS. Babies born to pregnant women who smoke have a higher risk of birth defects and low birthweight.

Until cigarettes were introduced in the early 1800s, tobacco was used primarily in the form of cigars, pipe tobacco, or snuff (a type of smokeless tobacco). The cigarette-manufacturing industry became a dominant force in the U.S. in the mid-1800s, at about the time of the Civil War. Various groups formed at that time to oppose smoking, but they disapproved of smoking because of moral concerns rather than health issues.

It was not until the early 1950s that smoking was first linked to the development of lung cancer, and in the next decade the Surgeon General's Office issued warnings regarding the dangers of smoking on health. In 1965 the U.S. Congress passed the Federal Cigarette Labeling and Advertising Act, which required the tobacco companies to place health warnings on all packages of cigarettes. Then in 1972 the Surgeon General issued a report that described the risk that SECONDHAND SMOKE posed to non-smokers.

In recent years the tobacco industry has faced increasing criticism over the health risks of tobacco, and many people have called for making the industry take greater responsibility for the health costs associated with their products. In 1994 Mississippi became the first state in the nation to sue tobacco manufacturers to recover costs for tobacco-related illnesses such as certain CANCERS and HEART DISEASE. Four years later the tobacco industry agreed to pay 46 states $206 billion as part of a major settlement of tobacco-related lawsuits against the industry. [*See also* TOBACCO AND HEALTH PROBLEMS; TOBACCO AND RESPIRATORY DISEASES; TOBACCO, FORMS OF; TOBACCO LAWS; TOBACCO SETTLEMENTS.]

TOBACCO ADDICTION Psychological and physical dependence on TOBACCO, which includes cigarettes, cigars, pipes, or SMOKELESS TOBACCO. Studies show that tobacco is as addicting a substance as HEROIN, COCAINE, and other highly addictive drugs.

HEALTH UPDATE

Smoking and the Grim Reaper
According to the CENTERS FOR DISEASE CONTROL AND PREVENTION (CDC), smoking kills more people every year in the United States than the combined deaths from motor vehicle crashes, AIDS, DRUG ABUSE, ALCOHOL ABUSE, Homicides, Suicides, and fires.

Keywords

bacteria microscopic, one-celled organisms that live both inside and outside the body, some of which can cause disease
nicotine a toxic and highly addictive drug found in tobacco

An estimated 66.8 percent of Americans over the age of 12 use tobacco, about 30 percent of the population of that age group. Moreover, studies show that tobacco use increases steadily during adolescence and early adulthood, from 2.2 percent of adolescents age 12 to 43.5 percent of individuals age 20. After age 25 tobacco use begins to decline due to SMOKING CESSATION or because tobacco users fall victim to the various diseases associated with tobacco use.

Most people addicted to tobacco are cigarette smokers (about 57 million Americans). However, a growing number also smoke cigars, which are the second most popular tobacco product. About 5 million people tried cigars for the first time in 1998, triple the number in 1991. The most popular forms of tobacco after cigarettes and cigars are smokeless tobacco (which includes chewing tobacco and snuff) and, finally, pipe tobacco.

Harmful Substances. Nicotine is the addicting substance in tobacco. A very fast-acting drug, it reaches the brain about ten seconds after a person inhales tobacco smoke. **Nicotine** acts as both a STIMULANT and a DEPRESSANT. As a stimulant, it causes higher levels of a brain chemical called *dopamine* to be released. This chemical affects the pleasure centers of the brain and also causes the heart to beat faster and blood pressure to increase. Yet nicotine can also act as a depressant, calming nerves and relaxing the muscles.

In addition to nicotine tobacco contains a number of toxic substances. Tar, a sticky residue from burning tobacco, sticks to the lungs where it traps **bacteria** and CARCINOGENS. This can lead to the development of such diseases as BRONCHITIS, EMPHYSEMA, and cancer. ***Carbon monoxide,*** an oxygen-robbing chemical present in the smoke generated by burning tobacco (see Volume 6), impairs the blood's capacity to carry oxygen, causing serious problems for people suffering from ***cardiovascular disease*** (see Volume 8).

Risks from Tobacco Use. According to the CENTERS FOR DISEASE CONTROL AND PREVENTION (CDC), 430,000 Americans die every year as a result of tobacco use. Regular use of tobacco dramatically increases the risk of a person developing some form of cancer, particularly LUNG CANCER. Tobacco products contain over 4,000 different chemicals, including 43 that are known carcinogens.

People addicted to tobacco also have a higher risk of respiratory diseases such as bronchitis, emphysema, and *pneumonia* (see Volume 8). Tobacco use contributes to HEART DISEASE, *stroke,* and *chronic obstructive pulmonary disease* (see Volume 8). Tobacco users also have higher rates of gastrointestinal disorders.

People addicted to tobacco endanger not only themselves but others as well. SECONDHAND SMOKE can be harmful to anyone who inhales it, and nearly a third of all children in the U.S. ages six and younger are exposed to someone who smokes inside the home.

Tobacco Users. Most people who become addicted to tobacco start smoking or using smokeless tobacco products during adolescence. Of adults in the United States who smoked at any time in their lives, 82 percent smoked their first cigarette before age 18. Of these more than half (53 percent) had become daily smokers before reaching their eighteenth birthday. Many teens do not believe they will become addicted to tobacco. Yet, although nearly half of those who use tobacco say they will not be smoking five years later, the majority of young smokers continue to smoke.

There are gender, racial, and educational differences among smokers. Males are more likely to smoke than females. In 1999, for example, 36.5 percent of all males ages 12 and over used tobacco products, compared to 24.3 percent of females in that age group. Males are ten times more likely than females to use smokeless tobacco, and they also lead in smoking cigars.

In terms of ethnic groups, Native Americans are the most likely of all groups to use at least one form of tobacco. Forty-three percent of Native Americans ages 12 and over smoke, followed by nearly 32 percent of whites and about 20 percent of African Americans.

Education is a significant factor in tobacco use, with more educated people less likely to use tobacco products. About 28 percent of college graduates smoke cigarettes, compared to 36 percent of individuals with some college, 42 percent of high school graduates, and about 47 percent of people without high school diplomas.

Ending Addiction. It is not easy to stop smoking because addiction to nicotine can be very powerful. However, it is possible and certainly advisable to kick the tobacco habit. There are a number of SMOKING CESSATION methods that can help people stop smoking. One method, NICOTINE REPLACEMENT THERAPY, involves the use of nicotine gum, skin patches, sprays, or inhalers. Another method involves use of a medication called Zyban (bupropion), which has been proven effective at helping people quit smoking.

Sometimes a combination of medications and individual *psychotherapy* or *group therapy* (see Volume 2) can be effective in smoking cessation. Some smokers have reported success with HYP-NOTHERAPY, while others have responded to *aversive smoking,* also called *rapid smoking,* in which people are told to smoke heavily and constantly (under supervision) until they become extremely nauseated and develop an aversion to tobacco. [*See also* DEPENDENCE, PHYSICAL; TOBACCO AND HEALTH PROBLEMS; TOBACCO AND RESPIRATORY DISEASES.]

TOBACCO ADDICTION, TREATMENT OF See NICOTINE REPLACEMENT THERAPY; SMOKING CESSATION; TOBACCO ADDICTION.

TOBACCO ADVERTISING See ADVERTISING AND MEDIA.

TOBACCO AND HEALTH PROBLEMS The links between TOBACCO and disease. A highly addictive substance, tobacco is responsible for more than 400,000 deaths in the United States each year, making it the leading cause of preventable deaths. Tobacco abuse also contributes to *cardiovascular disease* and to *chronic obstructive pulmonary disease* (see Volume 8) such as BRONCHITIS and EMPHYSEMA. Most people start using tobacco in their early teens, when it is difficult to foresee the damage that tobacco can cause to their bodies.

Of the approximately 57 million cigarette smokers in the United States many will eventually become ill with cancer and other diseases related to smoking, such as HEART DISEASE and *stroke* (see Volume 8). Chewing tobacco, a form of SMOKELESS TOBACCO, also presents various health risks, including ORAL CANCER, gum disease, and heart disease.

Cigar smokers have an even greater risk for heart disease than those who use smokeless tobacco. They also face a risk for lung cancer and oral cancer. This is cause for concern because cigar smoking nationwide increased by about 50 percent from 1993 to 1997. Many people may mistakenly believe that cigars are safe.

Cancer. Tobacco is known to cause a variety of CANCERS, including cancer of the lung, throat, esophagus, mouth, and bladder, and it is also associated with cancer of the stomach. Smokers who are deep inhalers have the greatest risk of developing lung cancer. Smoking is also a contributing factor to cancers of the kidney and pancreas, and it is suspected of contributing to colon cancer and liver cancer.

Cardiovascular and Respiratory Diseases. Smoking causes or contributes to both heart disease and stroke. Because smoking places a strain on the heart and blood vessels, it can lead to a

---

FEMALE VICTIMS OF TOBACCO DISEASES

Women smokers are at an increasing risk for the health consequences associated with TOBACCO, while the number of men smokers has declined. Between 1960 and 1990 the rate of death from LUNG CANCER increased by more than 400 percent for women. Why this dramatic increase? One reason is that during that time through ADVERTISING AND MEDIA many women were fooled by the tobacco companies into thinking that smoking was a liberating experience and made them more equal with men.

heart attack. Tobacco also increases blood pressure, furthering the risk for heart disease and stroke.

Illnesses such as ASTHMA, bronchitis, emphysema, and *pneumonia* (see Volume 8) are greatly worsened by smoking. Some older individuals who have smoked for many years often can breathe only with great difficulty and pain, and some must take supplemental oxygen in order to breathe.

Women and Smoking. For women smoking can damage the reproductive system, and it is associated with menstrual difficulties and fertility problems. It may also contribute to the early onset of *menopause* (see Volume 3). Smoking is harmful for the skin, causing for an early aging effect and deepening the fine lines around the mouth and eyes. Years of smoking tends to give the skin a leathery texture.

Cigarette smoke is classified as a **teratogen** because it poses a great danger to a developing fetus. For this reason, physicians advise all women who smoke to end their habit before getting pregnant as well as to avoid smoking during pregnancy and afterwards. Smoking during pregnancy can cause ***birth defects*** (see Volume 3), and it may result in infants born prematurely, of low birthweight, and at high risk for Sudden Infant Death Syndrome (SIDS), a tragic circumstance in which a newborn dies suddenly for no apparent reason.

Secondhand Smoke. Smoking affects not only the health of people who smoke but also others around them. Sometimes referred to as **passive smoking**, the inhalation of SECONDHAND SMOKE that is generated by smokers can cause lung cancer and respiratory ailments in others who share the same home or work environment. [*See also* PREGNANCY AND TOBACCO, ALCOHOL, AND DRUGS; TOBACCO ADDICTION; TOBACCO AND RESPIRATORY DISEASES.]

MORE SOURCES See www.cancer.org; www.lungusa.com

TOBACCO AND RESPIRATORY DISEASES Links between tobacco and various diseases of the respiratory system. Tobacco use is associated with a number of *chronic obstructive pulmonary disease* (see Volume 8). The primary cause of EMPHYSEMA, smoking also contributes to an increased risk for ASTHMA and BRONCHITIS. Smokers also have a greater risk than nonsmokers of contracting *pneumonia* (see Volume 8).

The chemicals in tobacco products harm and eventually destroy the microscopic hairlike cilia in the lungs, which provide protection against bacteria and other foreign invaders. Damage to the lungs allows CARCINOGENS to act against the body and cause CANCERS. Tar, a sticky residue from burning tobacco, and other unknown chemicals in tobacco can also affect the throat and lungs, causing a chronic severe cough. [*See also* TOBACCO AND HEALTH PROBLEMS; TOBACCO, CHEMICALS IN.]

TOBACCO CESSATION See SMOKING CESSATION.

TOBACCO, CHEMICALS IN Chemicals found in TOBACCO that can cause addiction or diseases such as CANCER. Tobacco contains over 4,000 different chemicals, at least 43 of which are known CARCINOGENS, or cancer-causing substances. The most prominent chemicals in tobacco are nicotine, tar, and *carbon monoxide* (see Volume 6).

Nicotine. Experts have called the cigarette a very efficient system for delivery of the drug nicotine, which is the addicting substance in tobacco. When a person uses tobacco, the nicotine is absorbed into the bloodstream and travels to the brain. The drug stimulates the brain, causing it to release adrenalin, which increases blood pressure and speeds up respiration and heart rate. Nicotine also causes the brain to release increased amounts of dopamine, a chemical that stimulates the pleasure centers of the brain. Individuals who smoke 30 cigarettes a day (a pack and half) will get 300 nicotine hits to their brain every day.

WITHDRAWAL from nicotine can be very difficult, and it takes at least several weeks before major withdrawal symptoms subside. For some people the craving for the drug persists as long as six months or more. Symptoms of withdrawal from nicotine include a continued craving for the drug, irritability, difficulty sleeping, problems keeping attention focused, and increased appetite. Many people who stop smoking gain weight because of increased appetite.

Toxic Substances. The two major toxic substances in tobacco are tar and carbon monoxide. Tar is a sticky residue from burning tobacco that can literally gum up the lungs, allowing bacteria and potential carcinogens to become trapped there. The buildup of tar can contribute to the development of LUNG CANCER or THROAT CANCER. It may also be a factor in the development of other diseases common to smokers, such as EMPHYSEMA and BRONCHITIS.

Carbon monoxide is a colorless, odorless gas found in the smoke produced from the burning of tobacco. An oxygen-robbing chemical, it impairs the ability of the blood to carry oxygen throughout the body and to the heart and brain. The carbon monoxide in tobacco can cause serious problems for people with *cardiovascular diseases* (see Volume 8). Its presence in SECOND-HAND SMOKE also poses a health threat to those around the smoker.

Smoking during *pregnancy* (see Volume 3) can be very harmful to the developing fetus. Exposure to carbon monoxide can result in infants born with low birthweights. Smoking during pregnancy may also contribute to birth defects such as cleft lip or cleft palate. Children born to women who smoke during pregnancy are also more likely to suffer from bronchitis, ASTHMA, and pneumonia, and infants are more likely to die from Sudden Infant Death Syndrome (SIDS), a tragic circumstance in which a newborn suddenly dies for no apparent reason. [*See also* PREGNANCY AND TOBACCO, ALCOHOL, AND DRUGS; TOBACCO ADDICTION; TOBACCO AND HEALTH PROBLEMS; TOBACCO AND RESPIRATORY DISEASES.]

TOBACCO, FORMS OF The different types of TOBACCO products. The most popular form of tobacco is the cigarette. In 1999, for example, about 57 million Americans smoked cigarettes. People also consume tobacco in the form of cigars, SMOKELESS TOBACCO, and pipe tobacco. About 12 million Americans smoked cigars in 1999, while 7.6 million used some form of smokeless tobacco, and about 2.4 million people used pipe tobacco.

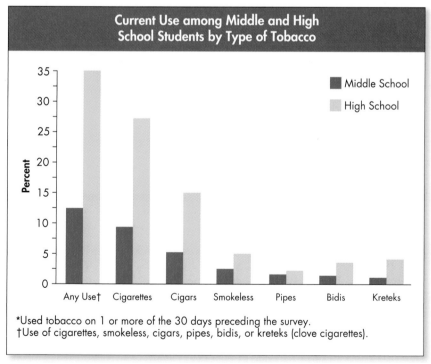

Current Use among Middle and High School Students by Type of Tobacco

*Used tobacco on 1 or more of the 30 days preceding the survey.
†Use of cigarettes, smokeless, cigars, pipes, bidis, or kreteks (clove cigarettes).

[Source: Centers for Disease Control and Prevention, National Youth Tobacco Survey, 1999.]

The tobacco for cigarettes and pipes is made from crumbled leaves. With cigarettes these crumpled leaves are put inside a thin paper wrapper. Pipe tobacco is loose and put into a pipe by the user. Cigars consist of whole tobacco leaves rolled tightly together.

Smokeless tobacco comes in several forms, which can be inhaled or chewed instead of smoked. One form of smokeless tobacco is snuff, a moist and finely ground powdered tobacco that is put into a nostril and inhaled or placed between the lower lip and gum, where it mixes with saliva. Chewing tobacco, which consists of more coarsely ground tobacco leaves, is held in the mouth between the cheek and gums. This "wad" or "chaw" of tobacco is then sucked and chewed. Chewing tobacco is also called spit tobacco because the user must frequently spit out the brown tobacco juice that forms as the tobacco is chewed.

TOBACCO LAWS State and federal laws that regulate the sale and use of TOBACCO in the United States. Tobacco laws in the U.S. are aimed primarily at protecting people from the harmful effects of smoking by controlling the sale and use of tobacco products. Some tobacco laws focus on attempts to prevent young people from smoking. For example, it is illegal in every state to sell tobacco products to individuals under age 18. However, enforcement of the law is more stringent in some states than in others.

Federal laws require cigarette manufacturers to place labels on every package of cigarettes warning consumers that smoking is dangerous to their health and may cause CANCERS and other diseases. Many states have also passed laws restricting the sale of tobacco in certain settings. For example, 41 states and the District of Columbia have some restrictions on cigarette sales through vending machines, and 19 states ban cigarette-vending machines in areas that are accessible to individuals under age 18.

Another way that government controls the consumption of tobacco is through excise taxes, which are taxes on particular products. All states have excise taxes on cigarettes, which raise the price of these tobacco products considerably. About half the states also have laws that restrict smoking at private worksites, either banning indoor smoking altogether or restricting smoking to special ventilated areas. Certain federal laws ban smoking on airline flights, while other laws prohibit smoking in certain public places such as movie theaters.

Provisions of State Laws Relating to Minors' Access to Tobacco as of December 31, 1999

State	Minimum age for tobacco sales	Tobacco license required	Vending machine restrictions	Enforcement authority	Sign-posting requirements*	Prohibits purchase, possession, and/or use by minors
ALABAMA	19	YES	NO	YES	NO	YES
ALASKA	19	YES†	YES	NO	YES	YES‡
ARIZONA	18	NO	YES	NO	NO	YES
ARKANSAS	18	YES	YES	YES	YES	YES
CALIFORNIA§	18	NO	YES	NO	YES	YES
COLORADO	18	NO	YES	YES	YES	YES
CONNECTICUT§	18	YES†	YES	YES	YES	YES
DELAWARE§	18	YES	YES	YES	YES	YES
DISTRICT OF COLUMBIA	18	YES†	YES	NO	YES	NO
FLORIDA§	18	YES	YES	YES	YES	YES
GEORGIA	18	YES	YES	YES	YES	YES
HAWAII	18	NO	YES	NO	YES	YES
IDAHO	18	NO	YESΔ	YES	NO	YES
ILLINOIS§	18	NO	YES	YES	NO¶	YES
INDIANA§	18	NO	YES	YES	YES	YES
IOWA§	18	YES†	YESΔ	YES	NO	YES
KANSAS	18	YES†	YES	NO	YES	YES
KENTUCKY§	18	YES†	YES	YES	YES	YES
LOUISIANA§	18	YES	YES	YES	YES	YES**
MAINE	18	YES	YES	YES	YES	YES
MARYLAND	18	YES†	NO	NO	NO	YES
MASSACHUSETTS§	18	YES	NO	NO	YES	NO
MICHIGAN§	18	YES	YES	NO	YES	YES††
MINNESOTA§	18	YES	YES	YES	NO	YES
MISSISSIPPI§	18	YES	YES	YES	YES	YES
MISSOURI	18	NO	NO	NO	YES	NO
MONTANA§	18	YES	YES	YES	YES	YES‡‡
NEBRASKA	18	YES§§	YES	NO	NO	YES
NEVADA§	18	YES§§	YES	YES	NO	NO
NEW HAMPSHIRE	18	YES	YES	YES	YES	YES
NEW JERSEY§	18	YES†	YES	YES	YES	NO
NEW MEXICO§	18	NO	YES	YES	YES	YES
NEW YORK§	18	YES	YES	YES	YES	NO
NORTH CAROLINA§	18	NO†§§ΔΔ	YES	NO	YES	YES
NORTH DAKOTA	18	YES§§	YES	NO	NO	YES
OHIO	18	YES†	YES	NO	YES	NO
OKLAHOMA§	18	YES†	YES	YES	YES	YES
OREGON§	18	NO	YES	YES	YES	YES
PENNSYLVANIA§	18	YES†	NO	NO	NO	NO‡‡
RHODE ISLAND	18	YES†	YES	YES	YES	YES¶¶
SOUTH CAROLINA§	18	YES	NO	NO	NO	NO
SOUTH DAKOTA§	18	NO	YES	YES	NO	YES

(continued)

Provisions of State Laws Relating to Minors' Access to Tobacco as of December 31, 1999

TENNESSEE§	18	NO	YES	YES	YES	YES
TEXAS	18	YES	YES	YES	YES	YES
UTAH§	18	YES	YES	YES	NO	YES
VERMONT	18	YES	YES	YES	YES	YES
VIRGINIA§	18	NO	YES	YES	YES	YES
WASHINGTON§	18†	YES†	YES	YES	YES	YES
WEST VIRGINIA§	18	NO	NO	YES	NO	YES
WISCONSIN§	18	YES	YES	NO	YES	YES
WYOMING§	18	NO	YES	NO	YES	YES
TOTAL	51	35	44	33	36	42

Except vending machines.
A retail license exists for those retailers who manufacture their own tobacco products or deal in nonpaid tobacco products.
On any public street, place, or resort.

*Refers to the requirement to post the minimum age for purchase of tobacco products.
†Excludes chewing tobacco or snuff.
‡Except minors at adult correctional facilities.
§Some or all tobacco control legislation includes preemption.
ᐃRequires businesses that have vending machines to ensure that minors do not have access to the machines; however, the law does not specify the type of restriction, such as limited placement, locking device, or supervision.
¶Signage required for sale of tobacco accessories, but not for tobacco.
**Except persons who are accompanied by a parent, spouse, or legal guardian 21 years of age or older or in a private residence.
††A pupil may not possess tobacco on school property.
§§Except vending machines.
ᐃᐃA retail license exists for those retailers who manufacture their own tobacco products or deal in nonpaid tobacco products.
¶¶On any public street, place, or resort.

[Source: Center for Disease Control and Prevention, Office on Smoking and Health, State Tobacco Activities Tracking and Evaluation System, unpublished data.]

TOBACCO SETTLEMENTS The results of large-scale lawsuits brought against the TOBACCO industry because of the health problems caused by tobacco. In the 1990s criticism of the tobacco companies for the role that tobacco played in health problems such as CANCERS and HEART DISEASE increased. Many people argued that the companies should bear some responsibility for the health costs associated with the use of their products.

In 1994 Mississippi became the first state in the United States to sue tobacco manufacturers in order to recover the costs for tobacco-related illnesses. The case was settled in 1997, and Mississippi set aside some of the funds from the settlement for use in tobacco control and disease prevention. After the success of the Mississippi lawsuit 46 other states sued the tobacco manufacturers.

In 1998 the tobacco industry as a whole agreed to a 46-state Master Settlement Agreement totaling about $206 billion to be paid over a number of years. As part of the settlement, the to-

Major Provisions of the Master Settlement Agreement

IN ADDITION TO THE MONETARY PAYMENTS FROM THE TOBACCO INDUSTRY TO STATES, THE SETTLEMENT PROVIDED FOR OTHER REQUIREMENTS AND RESTRICTIONS:

YOUTH ACCESS

- NO FREE SAMPLES EXCEPT IN AN ENCLOSED AREA WHERE OPERATOR ENSURES THAT NO UNDERAGE PERSONS ARE PRESENT.
- NO GIFTS TO YOUTH IN EXCHANGE FOR BUYING TOBACCO PRODUCTS.
- NO GIFTS THROUGH THE MAIL WITHOUT PROOF OF AGE.
- PROHIBITS SALE, MANUFACTURE, OR DISTRIBUTION OF CIGARETTES IN PACKAGES OF FEWER THAN 20 UNTIL DECEMBER 31, 2001.

MARKETING

- NO BRAND NAME SPONSORSHIP OF CONCERTS, TEAM SPORTING EVENTS, OR EVENTS WITH A SIGNIFICANT YOUTH AUDIENCE.
- NO SPONSORSHIP OF EVENTS IN WHICH PAID PARTICIPANTS ARE UNDERAGE.
- BANS USE OF TOBACCO BRAND NAMES IN STADIUMS AND ARENAS.
- BANS USE OF CARTOON CHARACTERS IN TOBACCO ADVERTISING, PACKAGING, AND PROMOTIONS.
- BANS PAYMENTS TO PROMOTE TOBACCO PRODUCTS IN ENTERTAINMENT SETTINGS, SUCH AS MOVIES.
- BANS DISTRIBUTION AND SALE OF MERCHANDISE WITH BRAND-NAME TOBACCO LOGOS.

LOBBYING

- PROHIBITS INDUSTRY FROM SUPPORTING DIVERSION OF SETTLEMENT FUNDS TO NONHEALTH USES.
- RESTRICTS INDUSTRY FROM LOBBYING AGAINST RESTRICTIONS OF ADVERTISING ON OR IN SCHOOL GROUNDS.
- PROHIBITS NEW CHALLENGES BY THE INDUSTRY TO STATE AND LOCAL TOBACCO CONTROL LAWS ENACTED BEFORE JUNE 1, 1998.

OUTDOOR ADVERTISING

- BANS TRANSIT AND OUTDOOR ADVERTISING, INCLUDING BILLBOARDS.
- TOBACCO BILLBOARDS AND TRANSIT ADS TO BE REMOVED.
- AT INDUSTRY EXPENSE, STATES COULD SUBSTITUTE ADVERTISING DISCOURAGING YOUTH SMOKING.

CESSATION AND PREVENTION

- THE TOBACCO INDUSTRY WILL CONTRIBUTE $25 MILLION ANNUALLY FOR 10 YEARS TO SUPPORT A CHARITABLE FOUNDATION ESTABLISHED BY THE NATIONAL ASSOCIATION OF ATTORNEYS GENERAL TO STUDY PROGRAMS TO REDUCE TEEN SMOKING AND TO PREVENT DISEASES ASSOCIATED WITH TOBACCO USE. THE FOUNDATION, SINCE NAMED THE AMERICAN LEGACY FOUNDATION, IS GOVERNED BY A BOARD AND WILL CARRY OUT A SUSTAINED NATIONAL ADVERTISING AND EDUCATION PROGRAM TO COUNTER TOBACCO USE BY YOUNG PEOPLE AND EDUCATE CONSUMERS ABOUT THE HEALTH HAZARDS OF TOBACCO USE. IT WILL ALSO EVALUATE THE EFFECTIVENESS OF COUNTERADVERTISING CAMPAIGNS, MODEL CLASSROOM EDUCATIONAL PROGRAMS, AND CESSATION PROGRAMS AND WILL DISSEMINATE THE RESULTS. OTHER ACTIVITIES INCLUDE COMMISSIONING AND FUNDING STUDIES ON THE FACTORS THAT INFLUENCE YOUTH SMOKING, DEVELOPING TRAINING PROGRAMS FOR PARENTS, AND MONITORING YOUTH SMOKING TO DETERMINE THE REASONS FOR INCREASES OR FAILURES TO DECREASE TOBACCO USE RATES.
- THE INDUSTRY WILL CONTRIBUTE $1.45 BILLION OVER FIVE YEARS TO SUPPORT THE NATIONAL PUBLIC EDUCATION FUND, WHICH WILL CARRY OUT A NATIONAL SUSTAINED ADVERTISING AND EDUCATION PROGRAM TO COUNTER YOUTH TOBACCO USE AND TO EDUCATE CONSUMERS ABOUT TOBACCO-RELATED DISEASES. THE TOBACCO INDUSTRY WILL CONTINUE TO CONTRIBUTE $300 MILLION ANNUALLY TO THE FUND AS LONG AS THE PARTICIPATING TOBACCO COMPANIES HOLD 99.05 PERCENT OF THE MARKET.

[Source: *Surgeon General's Report*, 1999.]

bacco industry also agreed in 1999 to remove all outdoor billboard advertising in the United States. Thirty-two of the states in the lawsuit have invested million of dollars from the settlement for use in tobacco prevention and control programs.

In addition to the Master Settlement Agreement three states besides Mississippi settled their claims individually with the tobacco industry: Florida, Texas, and Minnesota. In addition, in July 2000 a Florida jury awarded $145 billion in damages to sick Florida smokers, but the tobacco industry has appealed this verdict.

TOLERANCE, PHYSICAL A condition in which an individual needs greater amounts of ALCOHOL, DRUGS, or TOBACCO in order to obtain the same effects. When people develop tolerance to an addicting substance, their bodies adapt to the substance so that increasingly larger doses are needed to produce the desired effect. This increases the hazard of any undesired effects of the drug as well. There is often a fine line between tolerance and dependence—a condition in which individuals become so accustomed to using a drug that they cannot function without it.

People who develop a physical tolerance to drugs, alcohol, or tobacco may be able to function with the substance, but they will experience symptoms of WITHDRAWAL if they stop taking it. The symptoms of withdrawal vary depending on the substance. They may include sweating, nausea, vomiting, and mental confusion. In more extreme cases withdrawal can cause seizures, DELIRIUM TREMENS (DTs), and even death.

DETOXIFICATION—the process of eliminating an addicting substance from the body—can be very difficult and sometimes dangerous because of the withdrawal symptoms. For this reason anyone who wishes to stop using an addicting substance—whether alcohol, drugs, or tobacco—should get advice and help from a physician. Addicts withdrawing from drugs or alcohol, in particular, may need to enter a drug rehabilitation facility while undergoing detoxification.

The DRUG ENFORCEMENT ADMINISTRATION (DEA) provides information on the various drugs to which people can develop a physical tolerance. In addition to alcohol and tobacco, these drugs include MARIJUANA, COCAINE, HEROIN, AMPHETAMINES, BARBITURATES, METHAMPHETAMINE, and METHADONE. [*See also* DEPENDENCE, PHYSICAL; DEPENDENCE, PSYCHOLOGICAL.]

TREMENS See DELIRIUM TREMENS (DTs).

TWELVE-STEP PROGRAM Self-help program created by ALCOHOLICS ANONYMOUS (AA). Designed to help recovering alcoholics stay off ALCOHOL, the Twelve-Step Program serves as a model for many other similar programs, including Narcotics Anonymous. The program emphasizes that the addict is powerless over alcohol (or other addicting substance) and stresses the influence of a higher power and the incurable nature of ALCOHOLISM or ADDICTION. People learn to take responsibility for their actions and work through the twelve steps of the program in order to gain mastery over their fate by adopting a policy of ABSTINENCE from alcohol or drugs.

Joining a Program. People begin the Twelve-Step Program under varying circumstances. Some come to the program voluntarily or at the urging of family members or friends or because of recommendations by doctors or therapists. Other people enter Twelve-Step programs as a requirement from their employers because of problems with alcoholism or DRUG ABUSE on the job. Many people in jail or prison may be required to enter a Twelve-Step program as a condition of their sentence or of their parole or release.

The Twelve Steps. All Twelve-Step programs follow the basic 12 steps created by Alcoholics Anonymous. A summary of these steps is as follows.

The Twelve Steps of Alcoholics Anonymous

1. WE ADMITTED WE WERE POWERLESS OVER ALCOHOL—THAT OUR LIVES HAD BECOME UNMANAGEABLE.
2. CAME TO BELIEVE THAT A POWER GREATER THAN OURSELVES COULD RESTORE US TO SANITY.
3. MADE A DECISION TO TURN OUR WILL AND OUR LIVES OVER TO THE CARE OF GOD AS WE UNDERSTOOD HIM.
4. MADE A SEARCHING AND FEARLESS MORAL INVENTORY OF OURSELVES.
5. ADMITTED TO GOD, TO OURSELVES, AND TO ANOTHER HUMAN BEING THE EXACT NATURE OF OUR WRONGS.
6. WERE ENTIRELY READY TO HAVE GOD REMOVE ALL THESE DEFECTS OF CHARACTER.
7. HUMBLY ASKED HIM TO REMOVE OUR SHORTCOMINGS.
8. MADE A LIST OF ALL PERSONS WE HAD HARMED, AND BECAME WILLING TO MAKE AMENDS TO THEM ALL.
9. MADE DIRECT AMENDS TO SUCH PEOPLE WHEREVER POSSIBLE, EXCEPT WHEN TO DO SO WOULD INJURE THEM OR OTHERS.
10. CONTINUED TO TAKE PERSONAL INVENTORY AND WHEN WE WERE WRONG PROMPTLY ADMITTED IT.

(continued)

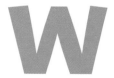

WINE See ALCOHOL.

WITHDRAWAL Process characterized by certain physical symptoms that addicts experience when they stop taking an addictive substance. The symptoms of withdrawal may be relatively mild, such as a headache, nausea, or general feeling of irritability. Withdrawal from TOBACCO generally produces mild symptoms. However, the symptoms of withdrawal may also be very severe. Withdrawal from long-term ALCOHOL ABUSE, for example, can cause DELIRIUM TREMENS (DTs) as well as seizures and HALLUCINATIONS.

Withdrawal from certain ILLEGAL DRUGS and prescription drugs can also produce very severe symptoms and be life-threatening. The symptoms of withdrawal from HEROIN include nausea and vomiting, profuse sweating, high fever, increased blood pressure and heart rate, tremors, severe joint and muscle pains, and convulsions. Withdrawal from BARBITURATES can produce nervousness, trembling, weakness, hallucinations, seizures, unconsciousness, and even death.

Because of the severity and potential danger of some withdrawal symptoms, physicians often recommend that people addicted to alcohol or drugs enter a hospital or special treatment center where medical staff can monitor them as they undergo the withdrawal process. Substance abusers may also be given medications to help reduce some of the physical effects of withdrawal. [*See also* ADDICTION; ADDICTION, STAGES OF; ALCOHOL ADDICTION; DEPENDENCE, PHYSICAL.]

Z

ZERO TOLERANCE LAWS State laws that designate very low limits of legal INTOXICATION levels for people under age 21. The legal limits of intoxication under zero tolerance laws differ depending on the state, ranging from BLOOD ALCOHOL LEVELS of just above zero to 0.02. By 1998 all states in the United States had enacted zero tolerance laws in response to passage of a federal law, the National Minimum Drinking Age Act of 1995. The aim of the laws has been to reduce injuries and deaths among adolescents caused by ALCOHOL ABUSE and DRIVING WHILE INTOXICATED OR DRUG IMPAIRED. [*See also* ALCOHOL LAWS.]

ZYBAN See ADDICTION, MEDICATIONS FOR; SMOKING CESSATION.

Concerns and Fears

Have you ever been afraid of something and then found out later that there was nothing to fear after all—like being afraid of the dark even though you really knew that you were safe and sound? Or have you ever done something without the slightest fear and then discovered that you were actually putting your life at risk—like stepping off a bus onto a busy street without looking? Both kinds of situations are very common, both can make you unhappy, and both can harm you either psychologically or physically. Having an exaggerated view of risks causes exaggerated fears, which can cause you to feel anxious and stressed out. Feeling this way for prolonged periods can make you physically ill. But having little or no concern about real risks can fool you into thinking that everything is fine when you are actually headed for major trouble. The stakes are especially high when the risks or fears involve your health.

Knowledge will empower you. Factual information about the true nature of the health risks associated with addictive substances can give you a more realistic perspective on them so that you can more accurately match fears with facts. You will then have a better chance to either feel better about the risks or at least be in a more favorable position to do something about them. The following are some examples of problems that are related to addictive substances and that many teens have to deal with as they get older and decide to use them or avoid them. Unfortunately, concerns about these issues are sometimes disconnected from reality. That is, in some cases, fears are often greater than the situation warrants, while in other cases, the risk seems to be hardly noticed at all. The following discussions may help put the problems in perspective.

ALCOHOL, DRUGS, AND INJURIES Because ALCOHOL and ILLEGAL DRUGS (as well as many prescribed drugs) can seriously impair the senses, this also means that they can greatly increase the risks to an intoxicated or heavily drugged person of getting hurt or dying in car crashes, water recreation accidents, fires, falls and other accidental injuries.

The normal reactions of individuals are delayed or impaired by alcohol or drugs. Or, they may be unconscious and completely unaware of harm that they may have inadvertently caused themselves or that is imminent, such as a fire caused by a dropped cigarette. In fact, the Centers for Disease Control and Prevention (CDC) reports that unintentional injuries are the cause of 60 percent of all adolescent deaths.

Car Crashes. The majority of teenage injuries are caused by car crashes, and teenagers are particularly at risk when they drive at night. Nighttime may be the "right time" to have plenty of fun when you are an adolescent, but unfortunately, it is also the time when many teens let down their guard, and they do not drive as well as they do during the day. It is also nighttime when teens are more likely to use drugs or alcohol. Another contributing factor to car crashes is that teens are less experienced drivers than most older people, and consequently they are also more likely to underestimate the risk of a dangerous situation. In addition, although teens do about 20 percent of all their driving at night, it is in the evening when half of all teenage driving fatalities occur.

Injuries that result from car crashes not only hurt or kill the person who is intoxicated or on drugs, but they harm many others as well. The CDC says that about 30 percent of all Americans will be involved in a car crash involving alcohol at least once in their lives, as drivers, passengers, or pedestrians. This percentage does not take into account the families of these individuals, who were not in the car or anywhere nearby, but who are terribly aggrieved by the injuries or deaths their relatives sustain from these crashes.

According to the CDC, alcohol is a factor in 35 percent of all adolescent driver fatalities. The CDC says that 21 percent of drivers ages 15–20 who died had blood alcohol levels above the legal limit for adults.

The CDC also reports that in 1998 teens represented about 10 percent of the entire population in the United States, but they accounted for 14 percent of all deaths in motor vehicle crashes. It is also true that when teenagers drive after drinking, they are more likely than adults to have a car crash, even when they have consumed less alcohol. Adolescent boys are at an especially high risk for having car crashes, and they have more than twice the risk of dying from car crashes as that experienced by teenage girls.

According to the CDC, other factors in car crashes in which alcohol abuse plays a role are poor driving decisions, such as choosing to run a red light or not stopping at a stop sign. Also, of all age groups who ride in cars, adolescents are the least likely to wear their seat belts. Yet simply buckling up the seat belt can literally mean the difference between life or death or between a severe or mild injury, should a car crash occur.

Drug Use and Risks for Injury. According to the CDC, DRUGS other than alcohol have been implicated in about 18 percent of the deaths of teenage drivers. Often the drugs of choice are MARIJUANA or COCAINE. Sometimes three or more drugs are used. Frequently, illegal drugs are combined with alcohol prior to the occurrence of injuries. Using both drugs and alcohol increases the risk of a car crash or other injury.

Drownings and Injuries in Water. Teens are also at risk for injuries and deaths that occur in the water (the oceans, lakes, rivers, swimming pools) and are related to alcohol consumption. For example, according to the CDC, in 40–50 percent of all adolescent male drownings, alcohol was involved. In general, the CDC says that alcohol is a factor in at least half of all the deaths of people of all ages that occur during water recreational sports.

Deaths or Injuries from Fires. Alcohol rears its ugly head yet again in deaths and injuries that result from fires that have their start in the home. The CDC says that alcohol is a contributing factor in 40 percent of such deaths. Smoking is the most common cause of deaths from fires that occur at home. It is not surprising that people who smoke and also drink are more likely to be very careless about the disposal of their smoking materials. Often, the intoxicated smoker simply falls asleep (or passes out) and then drops the cigarette on the floor. It then catches fire with something flammable. Because of their extreme intoxication, these individuals do not wake up in time to save themselves from the fire that they caused.

In one study that was performed in North Carolina on people who died in house fires, the researchers found that deaths were most likely to occur to males who were intoxicated and were at home by themselves. Others who were also at high risk were those who were impaired by both alcohol and drugs.

Another high-risk group was children under the age of five. In these cases children were either left alone or their caregivers were too intoxicated or drugged to save them in time from the fire. The children were too young to act to save themselves and their caregivers.

Falling Down. A fall is another category of injury that happens to many people who are impaired by alcohol or drugs. In fact, some people use the phrase "falling-down drunk" to refer to severe intoxication. When you are a teenager, such falls may cause no injury or they may lead to broken bones. When you are older, they may cause much more severe injuries. Of course, even an adolescent can be injured from a fall and can severely harm the brain or spine, causing traumatic brain injury or permanent paralysis. For example, an intoxicated or drugged teenager may not think about testing the depth of a creek and may leap into it, causing spinal damage that cannot be repaired.

At least 18 percent and as many as 53 percent of all nonfatal falls that occur in the U.S. are caused by excessive drinking. This is certainly a very wide range, but researchers say that the reason for this is that emergency rooms do not report the involvement of alcohol or drugs in their reports unless the person dies.

WOMEN AND THE RISKS OF ALCOHOL ABUSE It may sound very sexist, but the fact is that alcohol is not an equal-opportunity drug. Instead, and in many ways, alcohol can be more harmful to women than to men. For example, researchers have recently confirmed that female alcoholics are more likely to develop breast cancer, although they are not yet sure by what mechanism this is caused.

Women can also become intoxicated from smaller amounts of alcohol than men need to become drunk. A 2001 study in *Alcoholism:*

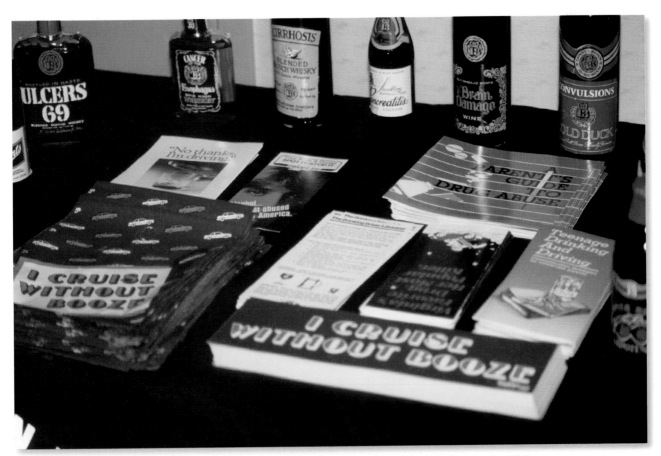
There are many programs that try to raise public awareness of the dangers of alcohol abuse and addiction.

Clinical and Experimental Research reported on a stomach enzyme, alcohol dehydrogenase (ADH), that is significantly less active in women and causes females to retain alcohol in their stomachs longer.

Interestingly, the metabolic difference between men and women was only found in forms of alcohol that had 10 percent or greater alcohol content. As a result, the researchers found that the female subjects metabolized BEER at about the same rate as men. However, because of the less-active ADH, when the female subjects drank stronger forms of alcohol, the alcohol remained in their stomachs for a period 43 percent longer than for the male subjects, speeding up intoxication.

Women generally also have more fatty tissue than males, which experts say may cause them to metabolize alcohol at a slower rate and thus become intoxicated more rapidly than men. According to the National Institute on Alcohol Abuse and Alcoholism, women generally have less body water than men, and this is yet another factor contributing to intoxication despite drinking less than men.

Women who become alcoholics are also more adversely affected by alcohol in some ways than are male alcoholics. For example, female alcoholics have a higher risk for CIRRHOSIS of the liver and alcoholic HEPATITIS. Researchers report that female alcoholics may also be more prone to brain damage from ALCOHOL ADDICTION than male alcoholics.

Female alcoholics have about the same risk as male alcohol abusers for heart problems, even though they usually drink significantly less alcohol. According to the National Institute on Alcohol Abuse and Alcoholism, women alcoholics have about a 60 percent lower lifetime alcohol use, despite the risk of heart problems that is equivalent to male alcoholics.

Breast cancer is another health problem faced by female alcoholics. Researchers in Canada found that women who drank the equivalent of four or five beers per day experienced 1.7 times the risk of nondrinkers in developing breast cancer.

Women who are heavy alcohol abusers are more likely than men to be physically or sexually abused by their partners or others. It is unclear whether this is because they are perceived as easy to abuse or if abused women turn to alcohol as an escape from early victimization in their lives. There may be other explanations as well.

Alcohol affects the reproductive systems of women and may cause irregular menstruation or infertility among heavy or alcoholic drinkers. Alcoholic women also have frequent difficulties in breast-feeding their infants (which may be a good thing for the babies, since they would be at risk of receiving alcohol from a drunken mother). If an alcoholic woman has a baby, her child is also at risk for FETAL ALCOHOL SYNDROME (FAS), which brings many lifelong medical and learning disabilities, such as development delays and mental retardation.

TOBACCO AND LUNG CANCER About 157,000 people in the United States die of LUNG CANCER every year; most of them started smoking when they were teenagers. About 80 percent of all lung cancers are caused by smoking. Smoking also causes other forms of deadly cancers, such as throat and mouth cancer or cancer of the esophagus (the food tube leading to the stomach). The reality is that even in our advanced high-technology society, we cannot always save people from severe illnesses. Yet it is also highly ironic when you think that lung cancer is the one disease that is almost always preventable, if only people would stop smoking.

Almost none of the people who die from lung cancer are teenagers. Instead, lung-cancer victims are usually middle-aged people like your parents or older people like your grandparents and other older relatives. Most people do not develop lung cancer until they are in their 40s or 50s, after many years of smoking. So if you smoke as a teenager, it is extremely unlikely that you will die from lung cancer in your teens. That will come later, assuming that you continue to smoke.

There are also some gender differences among those who develop lung cancer. According to the American Lung Association, male smokers are 22 times more likely to get lung cancer than men who are not smokers. Female smokers are 12 times more likely to get lung cancer than women nonsmokers. On the surface this might apear to mean that women are faring better than men on the issue of lung cancer. In general, this is true; however, the rate of lung cancer for men is dropping, while the rate for women with lung cancer is rising. Also, more women contract and die from lung cancer than women who develop breast cancer. Yet unlike breast cancer, lung cancer is preventable. There are many theories on why so many women are smoking themselves to death, such as targeted advertising by cigarette companies or social pressure that women today face.

It is also sad to think that many people who get lung cancer do so not from their own smoking but from SECONDHAND SMOKE that they are exposed to from others. Environmental tobacco smoke causes about 3,000 lung-cancer deaths per year among those who are nonsmokers. Many victims are children, who have no control over the smoking behavior of their parents or their parents' friends. Children who see their parents smoke are also more likely to smoke when they are adolescents, perpetuating the problem into the next generation. Secondhand smoke also causes heart disease and respiratory problems in others who do not smoke but who inhale the cigarette smoke of others.

ILLEGAL DRUGS AND MENTAL HEALTH

Some people worry that if they take an illegal drug, then it will affect their brain so much that they will become mentally ill and never recover. In most cases, even illegal drugs will not cause a person to lose touch with reality permanently, although temporary problems of rage or paranoia can often occur, sometimes with serious consequences. However, long-term (sometimes short-term) use of illegal drugs can lead to psychosis and serious psychological problems such as aggressive behavior or depression. Some drugs such as HALLUCINOGENS may trigger a mental illness in some people who are susceptible.

Most people use illegal drugs for their *psychoactive* properties, which means they use drugs to get high or to calm themselves down. Some people use hallucinogenic drugs such as LSD or PCP because they want to have an overall exciting experience or enhance a sexual experience. Researchers say that sex is not better with drugs such as PCP and that people who take these drugs are at high risk for heart attack and even death.

It is certainly true that people who use hallucinogens may have exciting HALLUCINATIONS, but often these hallucinations are unusually terrifying. People who use hallucinogens also experience terrifying "flashbacks," which are repeat hallucinations that occur long after the drug was used. Sometimes these drugs cause PSYCHOSIS.

Some drugs, such as METHAMPHETAMINE or ECSTASY, have been shown to cause brain damage among users, leaving them with memory problems, difficulty in thinking, and learning disabilities that were not there before the drug was used. This brain damage is permanent, even if the person never used drugs again.

Many drugs cause psychological problems. ANABOLIC STEROIDS can cause psychotic rages in users. Cocaine users may have extreme hallucinations—for example, that they are infested with insects that are either on or, even more frightening, underneath their skin. Cocaine users may also become psychotic. CRACK COCAINE can cause an extreme form of paranoia among users. Long-term alcoholism can cause psychosis and a form of dementia unique to alcoholics. The frequent use of marijuana can result in memory loss, difficulties in both problem-solving and thinking, and anxiety and panic attacks. Both the short- and long-term use of marijuana can cause anxiety, delusions and paranoia. Amphetamine use can incite an individual to violent behavior. Methamphetamine abuse causes memory loss, brain damage, hallucinations, paranoia, heart attack, and psychosis.

INHALANTS can cause brain damage and memory impairments. PCP may cause hallucinations, mood disorders, and amnesia, as well as a psychosis that is a virtual twin to schizophrenia, a severe mental illness in which the person has lost all touch with reality.

Addiction to Prescribed Drugs: OxyContin.

It is not only illegal drugs that are dangerously addictive. Some prescribed drugs may be addictive as well. Some adolescents mistakenly believe, however, that any drug that is prescribed by a doctor is also safe to abuse as a recreational drug. This is an extremely risky and wrong assumption.

According to federal government reports in 2001, the drug Oxycontin, which is an opioid painkiller, has become a drug of abuse among many people—and the abuse of this drug appears to be growing. The primary ingredient of OxyContin is oxycodone, which is also found in Percodan and other very strong pain medications. OxyContin is considered an effective drug for people suffering from cancer, serious injuries, or chronic and severe pain. It is a timed-release tablet that can provide pain relief for legitimate users for up to 12 hours. However, some abusers crush the tablet to enable them to get an instant "high." Adolescents and young people who are abusers also mix alcohol and illegal drugs with OxyContin, which may lead to death or serious illness.

According to the Center for Substance Abuse Treatment, when OxyContin is taken as directed, few users become addicted. For those who do develop an addiction, or for those who abuse the drug illegally and then become addicted, if they cannot obtain a legal prescription from a doctor, then they are at very high risk for stealing the drug or buying the drug on the street because the addiction is so strong. In addition, if these individuals find themselves unable to obtain OxyContin, they are at high risk for turning to heroin as a substitute drug. HEROIN is always illegal. Heroin is also dangerous because it is injected. The relative purity of heroin varies, and users also do not know what other substances may have been included in the drug. Many people who use heroin also share needles, and thus they are at high risk for contracting HIV, hepatitis, and other diseases that are transmitted through body fluids.

Because of the very powerful addiction that can occur from misuse of Oxycontin, experts say that it is too dangerous to simply stop taking the drug, because the person could become severely ill or die. For those patients who may legally take the drug, the first choice in getting off OxyContin is to taper it off slowly under medical supervision. Others who are addicted to this drug should receive medical treatment with either methadone or levo-alpha acetyl methadol (LAAM), both of which are treatment drugs used primarily for those with an addiction to heroin. Experts say that some addicts with very strong social supports may be able to resolve their addiction with the drug NALTREXONE.

Alcohol/Drug Use and Problematic Behavior.

Researchers have found many ties between the consumption of alcohol or illegal drugs and the subsequent commission of crimes or of serious problem behaviors such as engaging in unplanned sex or failing to use contraception. This is even true when it was the victim who was the one who had consumed alcohol or drugs.

In a 1997 survey of college students who were harassed or attacked, in the majority of cases the victims had used alcohol or drugs prior to the attack. For example, in the category of "unwanted sexual intercourse," in 82 percent of the cases, the victim had been using drugs or alcohol. In the category of "forced sexual touching or fondling,"

69 percent of the victims had used drugs or alcohol before the incident. For students who experienced physical violence, 69 percent of the victims had used drugs or alcohol beforehand. Apparently, people who abuse drugs or alcohol are easier to victimize by predatory individuals. It is generally much easier to attack a person whose senses are too impaired to run away or to think to scream for help from others.

Not surprisingly, those students who victimize others or behave in very destructive ways are also more likely to have abused drugs or alcohol. For example, adolescents who are ages 12–17 and use marijuana are more than twice as likely to attack other people, steal items, or vandalize and destroy the property of others. Among adults, alcohol is a factor in up to two-thirds of all murders, with either the perpetrator or victim (or both) drinking alcohol prior to the crime. In the cases of about 11 million victims of violent crime each year, about 3 million reported that the offender had been drinking alcohol before committing the crime. In addition, most experts implicate alcohol use by the offender in the majority of all sex crimes as well as crimes of child physical and sexual abuse.

In some cases "date rape drugs" that are tasteless, odorless, and difficult to detect with special laboratory screens—such as Rohypnol or ketamine—are purposely used by people who specifically plan to cause another person to unknowingly experience unconsciousness and amnesia. The unconsciousness enables the offender to sexually abuse the victim. The amnesia will prevent the victim from remembering the attack with any clarity, if at all.

It Can't Happen to Me

Like almost all teens, you probably feel pretty well most of the time. You rarely if ever think about what it would be like to be seriously ill or addicted to anything. Most of the really sick people you know are much older, and you are still young and healthy. Of course, you realize that teenagers can abuse or become addicted to drugs, alcohol, or tobacco, and that sometimes these things can cause serious and even life-threatening problems. But to you? Not too likely.

What if someday you did become a substance abuser? Or what if you only used a drug or alcohol once and there was a terrible consequence?

Most teens who discover that they have an addiction to alcohol, drugs, or tobacco are stunned and shocked. Often they truly cannot believe it. They feel scared, confused, and angry, and eventually they also feel depressed.

But most teens rise to the challenge and overcome the problems. They fight back. They adapt. They try to get the best medical care they can. They adjust to their new circumstances. They often overcome their abusive or addictive behavior and learn how to be happy and successful once again, despite it.

What is it like to be a teenager who has abused or is addicted to alcohol, drugs, or tobacco, and has suffered as a result? The stories that follow should give you some idea. All feature young people who, despite confronting some frightening problems, emerged stronger than before.

ALEISHA Sometimes the choices that you make in a very brief period can harm you and others for a long time. Aleisha, 14, was very jealous one night when her older brother Donny, 18, and his girlfriend Tracey, 17, were having a great time, drinking beers and laughing hysterically over everything. Aleisha wasn't in on any of the jokes and she didn't have a friend to talk to about it. "Everyone I knew was busy that night, and even Mom and Dad were out of town," recalls Aleisha.

She was lonely and bored and she didn't like how Donny and Tracey were acting at all. Aleisha also knew that her brother and his girlfriend were both underage for drinking, but that clearly didn't bother them at all, as they kept popping open more beers throughout the evening.

Aleisha decided that maybe she would have a few beers too. Why not, after all? There were plenty more beers in the fridge, and if those ran out there were lots of extra six-packs out in the garage. Aleisha had never tried any alcohol before, including beer—but it sure seemed to be making Donny and Tracey very happy. "I felt like I just had to do something or burst," says Aleisha.

So she walked over the refrigerator and pulled out a beer, popping it open for herself. Donny and Tracey noticed, but they didn't seem to care. Tracey said something like, "Yeah, you go girl!" although Aleisha's memory is not that clear about it. Soon Aleisha had consumed five or six cans of beer, as fast as she could drink them. She didn't like the taste at all, but she was determined to join in on the fun, whatever it took to get there. But drinking did not make things any better at all. Donny, pretty drunk himself, started calling Aleisha names, telling her she was fat and useless and that nobody, just nobody at all, in school liked her. She was a total loser. Her birth was probably an accident. And much more.

She is not even sure how it all happened so fast, but Aleisha remembers that at one moment, Donny was taunting her, and then the next minute she spotted a very large and very sharp butcher knife on the kitchen counter. Aleisha picked it up and she waved the knife threateningly at Donny, just to make him stop saying all those mean things. But this action only seemed to goad Donny more. He began shouting at her, "Go ahead, stab me! You can't do it, you're too afraid. Go ahead, go ahead, you're afraid, you're useless, you're stupid." He even ripped his shirt open and bared his chest, defying her to do anything.

In a fit of anger, Aleisha darted forward and stabbed Donny directly in the chest. Blood was suddenly everywhere and she heard herself screaming as Donny fell backward, at first moaning and then unconscious. She thought she had killed him. A sobbing Tracey called the 911 emergency number, and soon Donny was rushed off to the hospital. The police also arrived to question Aleisha and would not let her go to the hospital with Tracey and Donny. She later learned that she had just missed Donny's heart.

Fortunately, Donny survived and had a complete recovery. But life was not the same after the stabbing incident. Aleisha was placed in a juvenile detention facility for weeks until the court hearing. Her parents came to see her and both of them, even her Dad, cried and asked her why had she done this? She didn't know.

At the court hearing, a police officer testified about what happened, and a social worker gave a report on the family. She had come to the house several times and asked everyone in the family numerous questions for hours. She had also gone to the juvenile detention facility to question Aleisha. Now, weeks later, at the courthouse, Aleisha's parents each pleaded and begged the judge to let Aleisha come home.

It was Aleisha's first offense, but it was a very serious one, so it was not at all certain the judge would agree. But the judge did let her go home, after he outlined all sorts of conditions and rules that the social worker had set up for Aleisha. She would have to attend anger management classes. She would have to see a counselor. She would have to be part of family counseling.

When Aleisha went home and saw Donny for the first time since the assault, it was very hard. She had trouble looking at him. "He looked like he would never trust me again. And I didn't blame him," said Aleisha. "He shouldn't have

teased me like he did, but that was no reason for me to stab him, even though I was totally drunk."

Five or six beers and a lot of pent-up anger were all it took to bring Aleisha's world crashing around her and her family. If she had it to do over again, what would she do? "I would just tell Donny to shut up and go to bed! Being bored is way better than the awful stuff that happened to us all because I lost control from drinking," says Aleisha.

The counseling that Aleisha, Donny, and her parents received helped them resolve many festering issues about their relationships. Her parents realized they should have talked about alcohol long ago. They also know they should not have had such a large supply of beer on hand. They got rid of all of it.

Donny knows now that he was wrong to drink in front of Aleisha and to tease her. He has given up drinking for good, as has Aleisha. His girlfriend Tracey has also decided that alcohol is not worth it.

"Donny has forgiven me," says Aleisha. "My parents have also forgiven me." Aleisha says the hardest part was forgiving herself. "I did a terrible thing and I will never do anything like that again," she says. "I'm only a kid but I'm a kid who can't handle alcohol and I know it."

JIM Although he had used "weed" a few times, Jim, 15, did not see himself as a real "druggie." He did, however, have a few friends like Ryan who were regular users of marijuana and other drugs. On the three or four occasions when Jim had used marijuana, he got the stuff from Ryan. "He always had it or he knew where to get it, and everyone knew that," says Jim. He also knew that Ryan was headed for trouble. Several times Ryan had brought marijuana to school, although according to school rules, anyone caught with any drugs on campus would be expelled. All the students knew this rule because the school made them sign a statement about it when they registered for school. Teachers also reminded them about the rule, at least a few times a year.

"I knew about the drug policy," says Jim. "I just never paid that much attention to it, since I was not a crackhead or anything like that, so I figured it didn't apply to me."

Jim was startled one day when Ryan came rushing up to him. "He said he had a cop on his tail and I had to help him and hold something for him." Ryan thrust the "something" into Jim's hand and he was gone. It was a few joints of marijuana, which Jim hurriedly stuffed into his back pocket.

Both teens had failed to notice Mrs. Brown, who had seen the entire exchange. She came over to Jim and asked him what Ryan had given him. He hesitated, and she then demanded that he show her. So he pulled out the marijuana and, after she pressed him for an explanation, he told her what had happened.

Because of the zero-tolerance policy on drugs in the high school, Mrs. Brown reported the incident to the principal's office. The boys and their parents were summoned to the school for appointments the next day at different times with the principal and the teacher. A police officer would be there as well. They were not to go to any classes.

The atmosphere at that meeting was very tense, as Jim sat between his very upset mother and father. The principal was there, along with the assistant principal, Mrs. Brown, and the police officer. They asked Jim several questions and then asked Jim's parents if they were aware of the seriousness of the situation. They said they were. In fact, they were so stricken-looking that it almost looked like they, rather than Jim, were guilty.

What happened next really shocked Jim. The principal, Mrs. Long, announced that Jim would be expelled, just as Ryan had been expelled earlier that day.

Jim's jaw dropped open. What? Didn't Mrs. Long, Mrs. Brown, and the others believe that Jim had only held the marijuana for a minute or so? In fact, they said, they did believe him. But the punishment for illegal drug possession on school property was expulsion. There were no exceptions.

On the plus side (although there did not seem to be any pluses at all that day), the police officer said no charges would be pressed against Jim, although there had better not be a next offense. Also, it was a few weeks before the end of the school year, and since Jim was a good student, he would still pass the ninth grade. Ryan, on the other hand, was a very poor student and would have to repeat the grade. Neither boy would be allowed to complete any schoolwork for the final month of school or take their final exams.

Jim and his parents had some long chats about what you owe your friends and what you owe yourself and whether or not it is worth it to help someone who is breaking a law. They talked a lot about drugs and how much trouble they can get you into. Jim didn't want to risk his future and he decided to avoid marijuana—and Ryan—altogether. There were plenty of other ways to have fun and plenty of other kids to have fun with. For Jim there were no other offenses, and he completed high school with a good record.

"It was a painful lesson to be thrown out of school like a criminal," admits Jim. "But I knew the policy, and even though I guess I didn't really think it could affect me, it applied to me as well as anyone else. I was wrong."

TROY Troy, 14, started smoking a year ago. Some kids had dared him to try it, and then it just became a habit. He didn't really see what the big deal was, although it was kind of a pain to have to get someone to buy him cigarettes, since he was underage and had to use up all his lawn-mowing money to pay for them. He was also getting a little more winded and tired lately, and it was harder and took longer to do the work.

His parents didn't smoke, and they had made it clear that they did not approve of smoking. A few times Mom and Dad had found cigarette butts outside on the lawn and had questioned Troy about them. "I said it was my friends and I would clean up after them," said Troy. "When they asked me if I smoked, I said, 'of course not,' and they believed me."

One hot afternoon, after an especially hard day at school and a monster algebra test, Troy got home and no one was there. He decided he deserved a smoke. "I figured I could get rid of it by the time anyone came home," he recalls. So Troy pulled out his pack of cigarettes buried at the bottom of his backpack and lit up.

Suddenly, he heard someone pull into the driveway. "I thought it was my Mom," says Troy. He panicked, quickly crushing out the cigarette. Looking frantically around for a place to ditch it fast, he suddenly stuffed the cigarette butt under the sofa cushion. "I was sure it was out," says Troy. As it turned out, the car that Troy thought was his Mom's was really someone else, who was apparently lost and using the driveway to turn around. "I was disgusted at my freaking out over nothing. So I decided to just clear out," said Troy.

Troy came back a few hours later to see smoke pouring from his home and fire trucks everywhere. He heard a fireman say, "We haven't figured out yet why it started, but nobody was home. One of the neighbors called it in."

Troy gulped and tried to get back into the house, but the fireman held him back. "Wait until you get the all-clear from us," he said. "We're not done here yet." The fireman seemed to suddenly see Troy's stricken face and told him, "Don't worry, it looks a lot worse than it is. Your house will be fine."

There was some smoke damage to the house and the sofa where Troy had stuffed his still smoldering cigarette was destroyed. "I realized then that I was not as mature as I thought I was," said Troy. "I decided I better kick the habit before I caused any more harm to myself or anyone else."

Troy gave up smoking "cold turkey," which is pretty hard, even if you've only been addicted for a few months, as he was. But he succeeded, and he's glad he did. "I know people who tell me they started smoking as young as me, and now they're old and sick with cancer," said Troy. "I don't want to be like that. And I sure don't want to burn my house down!"

HOLLI Holli, 16, had never been to a rave before, and it sounded really exciting. "All-night music and dancing and plenty of guys—what could be better?" Holli remembers thinking at the time. Her pals Sandy and Colleen would be going with her, so everything should be okay. They had been to a rave a few months ago and said it was really amazing and she just had to go.

At the rave the music was deafening, and the atmosphere was charged with excitement and a feeling of defiance and high energy. Holli was definitely up for this. Then things got even better. She saw Sam, a guy in her history class, and waved at him. He pushed his way through the crowd to come over to her, and he asked Holli how things were going.

"You want to have a really good time, Holli?" Sam asked, talking so fast she could barely understand him. Sam held up a little white pill in the shape of a four-leaf clover. "You gotta try this," he said.

"What is it?" asked Holli. She had diabetes, and the only drugs she ever took were her insulin shots. She had taken a shot before she left home, so she felt good to go for the night.

"It's Ecstasy, babe! It is unbelievable! Just take one. It can't hurt you," Sam assured her.

Holli wasn't so sure about this. Her doctor had always warned her about taking any medications without checking with him first, because they might not go well with her insulin. But one little pill? Just one time? And besides, how could she say no to Sam, who was looking at her with such frank admiration? He would think she was immature if she turned him down. The admiring looks and the attention would be gone, and he'd move on to someone else.

"Well, maybe. But I'm not sure . . ." said Holli.

"Come on!" Sam said impatiently. "You haven't lived until you've tried this stuff. It'll be great, only happy times for you and me."

Holli liked the sound of the "you and me" part, so she took the drug from Sam and swallowed it down with her soda. She felt okay at first, but within an hour Holli's temperature shot up. She didn't know it, but her body temperature had soared from its normal temperature of 98.6° to an incredible 108°. "I felt terribly thirsty and terribly sick," recalls Holli. She tried drinking as much sugary soda as fast as she could, because Holli felt she was becoming dehydrated.

But she could not keep up with the effect of the Ecstasy. Somehow, with the help of her friends whom a now-concerned Sam had frantically flagged down, they got Holli outside where the air was cooler. It wasn't enough, and she passed out.

A scowling police officer came over, thinking it was yet another drunk or drugged-out underage kid he was seeing. But Sandy and Colleen knew that Holli had diabetes, and they told the officer. Holli also had an emergency medical bracelet that said she had "Type 1 diabetes" and required insulin. The bracelet had the name of her doctor too.

The police officer called in the emergency squad, and the still-unconscious Holli was rushed to the hospital in an ambulance, her anxious friends at her side. Was she going to die? Sandy and Colleen moaned to each other that it was all their fault. They should never have brought Holli to that stupid rave. Sam thought to himself that it was really his fault. He should never have given Holli that Ecstasy. But how was he to know Holli was diabetic?

All the teenagers were right. They were also wrong. Colleen and Sandy should not have encouraged Holli to go to the rave, knowing drugs were everywhere. They shouldn't have gone there themselves either. Sam was also right. He should never have given Holli the Ecstasy. However, even if Holli didn't have diabetes, she still could have become extremely sick, and even died, from one dose of the drug.

At the emergency room the staff shooed away the teens into the waiting room as they worked on Holli. Sam got a message to the doctor that Holli "might have" taken some drug like Ecstasy. The ER doctor decided he had to pump the drug out of Holli's stomach, so he inserted a tube down the unconscious girl's throat. The stomach pump would get rid of the drug as quickly as possible.

The ER staff also started an intravenous tubing on Holli and administered glucose to counteract the hypoglycemia she was experiencing. Even though diabetes is a condition of excessively high glucose, or "sugar" (hyperglycemia), sometimes the levels can go too far in the other direction, and the diabetic person actually needs glucose to live. That is what happened to Holli because of the hyperthermia and dehydration induced by taking Ecstasy.

"I woke up in the hospital emergency room, and I didn't know where I was or what happened," recalls Holli. She had a splitting headache, and her throat hurt from the stomach pump. But she was alive, and the doctors found no permanent damage. They issued her a very stern warning. "The doctor said I nearly died of a drug overdose," says Holli, her eyes filling with tears. "It wasn't worth it! I will never do anything like that again!"

Straight Talk

To some questions that you ask, you can expect honest answers. What time does the movie start? How much does that job pay per hour? But the facts often fly out the window when you ask a question about which people have strong opinions. What's wrong with trying cigarettes just once? Does everyone who tries drugs become an addict?

Some people who give biased answers to teens' questions think that they know what is best for the teen, and the facts do not really matter as much as steering a teen in the "right" direction. Say that you ask an adult about almost anything to do with drugs. Or sex. Maybe the adult thinks that using drugs in the teen years is wrong because they're bad for the body or because they're illegal. Maybe the adult thinks sex in teen years is never safe because teens are not mature enough to handle the possible consequences, or maybe the adult opposes sex before marriage. The answers you receive in these cases are likely to skew the facts in the direction that the adult wants your behavior to go.

Here you will find straight answers to some common teen questions related to addictions to alcohol, drugs, and tobacco, based not on biases, but on the best information available—not on opinion or emotion but instead based on facts.

WHY CAN'T I JUST TRY SMOKING ONCE? NOT EVERYONE GETS ADDICTED, DO THEY?
No, not everyone who tries a cigarette for the very first time will then automatically become a regular or heavy smoker for years. But the reality is that many people who try smoking for the first time *do* become addicted to TO-BACCO, and they continue to smoke for many years or even for the rest of their lives. At the same time, it is also true that there are other people who try smoking one time, and then they never smoke again.

It is very hard to predict if a person will be one of the many people who start smoking and then become addicted. It is also hard to predict if, instead, the teen experimenting with tobacco will be among those who do not smoke again. What we do know for sure, however, is that virtually everyone who starts smoking is convinced that they could give up the habit whenever they want to. Sadly, once you are addicted to tobacco, it is far more difficult to quit smoking than many teenagers realize. Also, most adults who smoke say, often with regret, that they started smoking as young teenagers.

Another thing you can know for sure about smoking is that the health risks for those who continue to smoke are very high. Experts report that smoking is the one preventable cause of illness or death from cancer, stroke, heart attack, and asthma—to name just a few of the many diseases that tobacco use can lead to. Yet largely because nearly all of these serious diseases are so far off in the distant future for teenage smokers, they don't worry about such illnesses or even think about these health risks.

Still, many teen smokers do have some early-warning health indicators of such problems to come, such as a hacking cough and a major mucus buildup as well as nicotine-stained fingers. Also, the urgency to smoke constantly is another indicator of a serious addiction to tobacco. Some people have to light up first thing in the morning and then have one last cigarette before they go to bed. For such people, that first cigarette is the best one—the one with the strongest "kick," since they have not had any nicotine all night.

What if you still want to try smoking, even after knowing about the many negatives associated with tobacco use? What are some of the odds of addiction? Here are the facts that we do know. Federal researchers reported in 1998 that about 36 percent of all kids ages 12–17 have tried cigarettes at some point in their lifetimes. Of these adolescents, about 18 percent say that they are either regular (about a pack a day) smokers or heavy users (more than a pack a day). Other studies looking at larger groups have found an even higher rate of addiction. For example, a 1994 study of tobacco use found that about one-third of tobacco users ages 15–24 become addicted to tobacco.

So if you decide to try smoking, you might be one of the people who smoke a cigarette once or twice and then never or very rarely smokes again. On the other hand, you could end up with a heavy smoking habit just as easily.

A major point to keep in mind when you consider experimenting with smoking is that tobacco is an extremely addictive drug. The physical addiction stems from the action of nicotine on the brain. Each time the smoker inhales the smoke, within about ten seconds a "hit" of nicotine surges to the brain, causing a variety of brain chemicals to react and the blood pressure to rise, creating multiple effects on the brain and the rest of the body.

The frequency of smoking is also a factor in continuing the addiction. The more times that people smoke, the more they become heavily dependent on those regular nicotine hits. Without the drug they feel tired, depressed, and deprived. People who have smoked for years *can* quit—with a major effort. It's just that it is even harder to quit after so many years of addiction.

There are some groups of people that are more or less at risk to continue smoking. For example, if you are Asian American or African American, you have less of a risk for becoming a smoker than the risk faced by whites, Hispanics, or Native Americans. But you are still not "safe" from developing an addiction. The only people who are safe from TOBACCO ADDICTION are those who do not smoke at all.

WHAT IF MY FRIENDS AND I SMOKE—BUT I WANT TO QUIT?

Another aspect of smoking which keeps many people using tobacco, or that makes them relapse after they try to quit, is that smoking is also a social activity. Males may have initially perceived smoking as a masculine or "male bonding" kind of activity. Young women may have viewed smoking as something glamorous that adult women do and that they would like to do with their friends.

Some people make a ritual of lighting up and smoking with their friends. If you start smoking with your friends who are already smokers, it can be hard to stop, because your friends are unlikely to want to quit at the same time. You will probably also find that it's hard to avoid smoking when you are around friends and family members who continue to smoke in your presence.

If you decide to quit smoking, it is a good idea to ask your smoking friends and family members to avoid leaving cigarettes lying around within easy reach. Those cigarettes could tantalize you, and you might even pick one up without thinking. When they are out of sight, cigarettes may not be entirely out of your mind, but it's still easier if you cannot see them right in front of you. Ask friends and family members who smoke if they could either not smoke or at least smoke less often when you are around. They may say no. But hopefully, they will respond to your very reasonable request.

After you have stopped smoking for a while, you may find that tobacco smoke bothers you and that you don't like the smell of tobacco smoke on your clothes or in your hair. You may also start encouraging your friends to smoke outside your home, if they can't or won't kick the habit.

Another good idea to help you stop smoking is to join with others who are also working to quit. Ask your doctor for the name of a smoking cessation group or contact the nearest hospital about whether they have any similar programs. Such programs offered by hospitals are often either free or inexpensive.

WILL I GET FAT IF I QUIT SMOKING?

Some people, especially adolescent females, worry that they will gain a lot of weight if they stop smoking. They imagine themselves becoming bloated to huge proportions. This fear looms so large in their minds that the many reasons to stop smoking are not important to them. To avoid this perceived risk of getting fat, they decide that they will just keep on smoking. Some experts report that white teenage girls are particularly susceptible to the fear of getting fat to keep them from stopping smoking. Researchers cite studies indicating that African American women are not as worried about this issue, perhaps because they are more secure in their body image.

Cigarette companies are very keyed in to this weight-gain fear among women, which is why they use words like "slim" and "thin" in the names of their products. It is also why cigarette advertisers use very slender or anorectic-looking models in their advertisements.

It is true that many smokers gain a few pounds when they stop smoking, as they learn to adapt to a nonsmoking lifestyle. However, the common fear of impending obesity is largely unfounded, according to the Centers for Disease Control and Prevention (CDC). They report that the average weight gain experienced by people who quit smoking is only about 5 pounds, and it can be controlled through exercise and diet. Some studies also indicate that nicotine replacement medicines or antismoking medications can also limit weight gain.

A weight gain may occur right after stopping smoking. But if you gain 3–4 pounds the first week that you quit smoking, don't panic and assume that this kind of weight gain will continue every week. Most of that weight gain in the first week is due to temporary water retention, which will go away once your body adjusts to not smoking.

Experts also report that people who have smoked for 10–20 years are the *most* likely to gain more than just a few pounds. However, this is not a problem for teens, because a 15-year-old would have had to start smoking at age five for this factor to matter. As a result, teenagers are less likely to gain weight than adults who have been smoking for years and then quit. However, if you wait until you are 30 or 35 years old (or older) to quit smoking, you might pack on the pounds at that time. Better to quit now and be ahead of the game.

It is also true that lighter smokers are less likely to gain weight. Some people, especially heavy smokers, gain more than 5 pounds and may increase their weight by as much as 7–10 pounds.

To avoid weight gain when you stop smoking, experts recommend that you drink plenty of fluids (rather than the sugary foods you may be drawn to), and especially drink plenty of water. Try to avoid caffeinated drinks such as colas, because they may boost your desire to both smoke and eat.

Don't skip meals when you stop smoking in an effort to keep your weight down. If you feel intensely hungry from trying to not eat, you may find yourself splurging on junk food and snacks. It's okay to eat cake or ice cream once in a while, as long as it's not an everyday occurence. It's best to go heavy on salads. You can also chew sugarless gum to control the desire to have something in your mouth.

It is also best to make a plan ahead of time for what you will do when the nicotine craving hits or you feel an attack of the "munchies." Experts report that those who avoid weight gains after quitting smoking are successful at finding other ways to distract themselves. When nicotine or food cravings hit you, go talk to a friend, go for a walk, or find something else to do!

To stay off cigarettes, it is also advisable to change your habits. Often smokers have behavioral "cues" that they link to their smoking. If you alter your habits, you can eliminate many of these cues, and often this will help you avoid both smoking and overeating. For example, if you always smoked after dinner at 6 P.M., then eat at a different time. Also, eat in a different place. Instead of eating and then smoking in front of the television (which is a bad idea for anyone, because it's too easy to overeat), sit down at a table and eat your food. Another example: If you always had Danish, coffee, and a cigarette after school, substitute another activity that is fun.

Stress can also cause you to smoke and overeat. If you feel stressed out, take a shower, listen to music, go for a walk or talk to a friend. Find a healthful and fun substitute activity.

IF MY PARENT IS AN ALCOHOLIC, WILL I BECOME ONE TOO? If you have a parent who regularly abuses alcohol or is addicted to it, then your risk for this behavior is greater than if your parent did not drink at all. There are gender differences, however. The risk for ALCOHOLISM is generally much higher for males than females.

Scientists have relied heavily on twin or adoption studies to try to determine the influence of nature (genes/heredity) versus nurture (environment). Identical twins share a genetic heritage, so if one twin becomes an alcoholic, then the other twin usually has an increased risk for alcoholism too. But there is still an environmental impact with twins, because they are usually raised together and thus share a common environment. In general, scientists believe that, based on the twin studies, at least half of alcoholism among males can be attributed to heredity. However, the genetic link between parents and daughters is not as clear-cut. Some researchers, however, argue that about two-thirds of the cause of alcoholism is due to genetics.

Scientists in Sweden, Denmark, and other countries have used adoption studies to help them evaluate the impact of heredity on social problems such as alcoholism. They have looked at adults who were adopted as children. The researchers compared the drinking behavior of these adults to that of their biological parents.

These studies have shown that the Scandinavian adopted men had a higher risk for becoming alcoholic if a birth parent was an alcoholic. The risk for alcoholism was far lower for female adoptees. (It is unclear whether this gender difference is a cultural or a genetic issue. Perhaps women are expected to drink less than men or perhaps they are genetically programmed to drink less. The research continues.)

The adoption-study researchers found that when neither biological parent was an alcoholic, then about 15 percent of the male adoptees were alcohol abusers (and 85 percent were not alcoholics). If only the birth father was an alcoholic, the percentage of male adoptees with alcohol abuses problems rose to 22 percent. If both birth parents were alcoholics, then about 33 percent of the adopted men became alcoholics. (This also means that 77 percent did not become alcoholics.) Thus, the genetic risks for adopted men to be alcoholic were highest when both birth parents were alcoholics.

Some studies have also looked at the adoptive parents and compared them to the adopted children. Very few adoptive parents are alcoholics, since they are carefully screened before they are allowed to adopt a child. However, the Scandinavian adoption researchers did find some adoptive fathers who were alcoholics. In those cases the risk for the adopted child becoming an alcoholic was greater than when the adoptive parent was not an alcoholic. If the biological father as well as the adoptive father was an alcoholic, the risk was even greater. This finding indicated that both environment and heredity affected the adoptee's behavior.

The linkage between the alcoholism of their birth parents and their own alcohol abuse as adults was much weaker when the researchers studied adopted women. They found that when the birth mother was an alcoholic, then about 10 percent of the female adoptees became alcohol abusers. If the birth mother was *not* an alcohol abuser, then only about 3 percent of the female adoptees became alcoholics. Whether the biological father was an alcohol abuser or not did not make any difference to the outcome of the adopted women.

Researchers have also found a significant relationship between adopted siblings and their drinking habits. If two unrelated children are adopted into a family, and one becomes a heavy drinker as an adolescent, the other child is more likely to become an alcohol abuser too, even though there are no shared genes between the two children. Thus, environment clearly plays a role in alcohol abuse too.

What about the actual genetic location of an "alcoholic gene?" Is there such a thing?

Researchers are trying to find the genetic location of a risk for alcoholism.

Interestingly, some scientists have apparently found an antidrinking gene. In the year 2000, genetic scientists found a gene, ADH2, that may protect against alcoholism. So far, the gene has primarily been found among people of Asian heritage. Research continues to determine if others may have protective genes.

Some scientists believe that it is not a tendency to alcoholism that is inherited but rather a tendency toward impulsive and/or addictive behavior that may be genetically based. If this is true, it explains why most alcoholics are also very heavy smokers.

So, bottom line, if one of your parents is an alcoholic, your risk for alcoholism is higher than if your parent did not drink. But you are not doomed to a life of alcoholism. Should you discover that it is difficult for you to stop drinking, it is best to keep the genetic risk in mind and forego alcohol. Some children of alcoholics choose to never drink, so that they can avoid any risk altogether.

WHAT IF ALL MY FRIENDS USE ILLEGAL DRUGS?

If all your peers are regular illegal-drug users, and you have so far avoided using illegal substances, it's probably a good idea to think about whether these friends are really worth your time and attention. Many of them will end up in jail or in psychiatric hospitals. They may wind up very sick or dead from drug-related ailments. No one wants these bad things to happen to their friends, but there is really very little you can do about it. You can talk about the evils of drugs to them, but if they are addicted your words are wasted. They will not listen.

Fortunately, most teenagers do not use illegal drugs, and you can work at befriending these teens. Find them in school, houses of worship, and special-interest clubs. For example, if you love swimming, which would be better to do: hang out with other swim freaks or with kids who live only for their next hit of cocaine? You know the answer to that one.

If you don't know how to find people who share your interests, contact your guidance counselor, read the local newspaper, or ask around. Eventually, and probably a lot faster than you can imagine, you'll find groups of kids who share common interests with you.

Will they be a little leery of you at first, knowing that you used to hang out with the druggies? Sure, they might be wary of you at first. But you can tell them up front that you are not and were not a drug user and you live to _____ (whatever activity they engage in). Pretty soon your enthusiasm and obvious sincerity will win them over.

IF I EAT A BIG MEAL AND DRINK LOTS OF COFFEE, COULD I STILL GET DRUNK?

Yes, you can still get drunk, even if you eat a lot of food and drink a lot of coffee. In fact, you could eat a five-course meal and still become intoxicated if you drank enough alcohol. It is true that someone who has not eaten much can become a little drunk faster than someone who eats a full meal, because food slows down the absorption of alcohol. But it is also true that consuming food does not convey automatic protection from drunkenness.

Contrary to popular belief, caffeine won't protect you from intoxication, nor will it help sober you up quickly once you are drunk. Caffeine may make you less likely to fall asleep after drinking alcohol, because caffeine is a stimulant. The old saying about coffee making a person a "wide-awake drunk" is actually quite true. Never assume that it is a great idea to urge an intoxicated person to drink cup after cup of coffee before he drives off. Better to take the car keys away from him and maybe save his life or the lives of others on the road.

Another reason why food cannot protect you from drunkenness if you drink too much is that the liver can only process so much alcohol at a time. So if a person pours on the alcohol, taking drink after drink, then that person will become intoxicated, regardless of how much food he or she has consumed. Another problem that can occur if people consume a full meal before drinking heavily is that excessive amounts of alcohol will usually upset their stomachs. They will often vomit!

WHAT IF MY BOYFRIEND OR GIRLFRIEND SAYS IF I REALLY CARED, I WILL TRY DRUGS TOO? This is a very old and tired argument that has been used in so many different ways by countless people who want to manipulate others. If you really care about them, or so these manipulative people say, then you will take drugs, have sex with them, or do something else that they want you to do. The manipulative person may try a variety of other arguments, such as telling you that you are acting like a little girl or boy because you refuse to give in.

The reality is, if the other person really cares about you, then he or she will accept "no" as the answer to the request—and leave it at that. If they do not, as difficult as it may be, you should move on. This is easy to say and hard to do. But it is a better choice than to allow yourself to use drugs or make other dangerous choices that could ruin your life, long after the person who encouraged you to try them is gone.

ARE PRESCRIBED DRUGS ALWAYS SAFE? Because prescription drugs are ordered by a doctor, some people think that they are safer than illegal drugs such as cocaine, heroin, or Ecstasy. While this is generally true, there are three important points to keep in mind. First, the prescribed drug needs to be taken as directed by the doctor, not more frequently or in larger doses.

Next, some drugs, even when they are used as directed, can become addictive. This is particularly true of some very strong painkilling drugs such as OxyContin, which most doctors now only prescribe for people with cancer. According to experts, OxyContin is stolen from pharmacies or from patients taking the drug, because the urge to abuse it is so strong. Other drugs, such as Percocet or Vicodin, are also prescribed drugs that are often abused.

Finally, drugs should be used only by the person for whom the doctor prescribed them. What may work very well for one person's body could be a drug that is toxic or fatal for someone else. It does not matter if the person with the prescription medicine is your parent or your sister. You could have a very different reaction to the medication than they would have. For example, you might have an allergic reaction. Thus, you should never take their prescribed drugs. In fact, it is illegal for anyone to give you their prescribed medicines.

LAST WORDS. Along with your sharp mind, your sense of humor, and your good looks, your health is often very easy to take for granted. But if you begin to suspect that something is not quite right with your body, or that taking actions such as trying alcohol, tobacco or drugs could possibly be risky, do yourself a favor. Instead of ignoring your own nagging questions, talk to someone who can give you the straight facts.

Directory of Services, Organizations, Help Sites, and Hotlines

Services and Organizations

For Volume 1: *Addiction: Tobacco, Alcohol, and Other Drugs*

American Cancer Society
1599 Clifton Road, NE
Atlanta, GA 30329
(800) ACS-2345
www.cancer.org

American Lung Association
1740 Broadway
New York, NY 10019
(800) 586-4872
www.lungusa.com

National Institute on Alcohol Abuse and Alcoholism
National Institutes of Health
6000 Executive Boulevard
Bethesda, MD, 20892-7003
(301) 443-3860
www.niaaa.nih.gov

National Institute on Drug Abuse
National Institutes of Health
6001 Executive Boulevard, Room 5213
Bethesda, MD 20892
(301) 443-1124
www.nida.nih.gov

Partnership for a Drug-Free America
405 Lexington Avenue, 16th Floor
New York, NY 10174
(212) 922-1560
www.drugfreeamerica.org

For the Set

American Academy of Family Physicians
11400 Tomahawk Creek Parkway
Leawood, KS 66211-2672
(913) 906-6000
www.aafp.org

American Academy of Pediatrics
141 Northwest Point Boulevard
Elk Grove, IL 60007-1098
(847) 434-4000
www.aap.org

American Medical Association
515 North State Street
Chicago, IL 60610-4377
(312) 464-5000
www.ama-assn.org

American Medical Women's Association
801 North Fairfax Street, Suite 400
Alexandria, VA, 22314
(703) 838-0500
www.amwa-doc.org

American Red Cross
431 18th Street, NW
Washington, DC 20006
(202) 639-3400
www.redcross.org

Association for the Care of Children's Health
19 Mantua Road
Mt. Royal, NJ 08061
(609) 224-1742
www.acch.org

Centers for Disease Control and Prevention
1600 Clifton Road
Atlanta, GA 30333
(404) 639-3311
www.cdc.gov

National Center for Health Education
72 Spring Street, Suite 208
New York, NY 10012
(212) 334-9470
www.nche.org

National Health Information Center
Office of Disease Prevention and Health Promotion
P.O. Box 1133
Washington, DC 20013-1133
(800) 336-4797
www.health.gov/nhic

National Institutes of Health
9000 Rockville Pike
Bethesda, MD 20892
(301) 496-4000
www.nih.gov

Office of Alternative Medicine
National Institutes of Health
9000 Rockville Pike
Bethesda, MD 20892
(888) 644-6226
http://nccam.nih.gov

Office of Minority Health Resource Center
P.O. Box 37337
Washington, DC 20013-7337
(800) 444-6472
www.omhrc.gov

U.S. Department of Health and Human Services
200 Independence Avenue, SW
Washington, DC 20201
(877) 696-6775
www.os.dhhs.gov

U.S. Food and Drug Administration
5600 Fishers Lane
Rockville, MD 20857-0001
(888) INFO-FDA
www.fda.gov

World Health Organization
CH-1211
Geneva, Switzerland
www.who.ch

Help Sites and Hotlines

For Volume 1: *Addiction: Tobacco, Alcohol, and Other Drugs*

Al-Alon and Alateen
1600 Corporate Landing Parkway
Virginia Beach, VA 23454
1-888-4AL-ANON
www.al-anon-alateen.org

Alcoholics Anonymous World Services
475 Riverside Drive
New York, NY 100115
1-212-344-2666
www.alcoholics-anonymous.org

Cancer Hope Network
2 North Road
Chester, NJ 07930
1-877-HOPENET
www.cancerhopenetwork.org

Cocaine Anonymous World Services
P.O. Box 2000
Los Angeles, CA 90049-8000
1-800-347-8998
www.ca.org

Marijuana Anonymous World Services
P.O. Box 2912
Van Nuys, CA 91404
1-800-766-6779
www.marijuana-anonymous.org

Narcotics Anonymous World Services
P.O. Box 9999
Van Nuys, CA 91409
1-818-773-9999
www.na.org

National Association for Children of Alcoholics
11426 Rockville Pike, Suite 100
Rockville, MD 20852
1-800-359-COAF
www.health.org/nacoa

National Council on Alcoholism and Drug Dependency
12 West 21st Street
New York, NY 10010
1-800-NCA-CALL
www.ncadd.org

National Heart, Lung, and Blood Institute Information Center
National Institutes of Health
P.O. Box 30105
Bethesda, MD 20804
1-800-575-9355
www.nhlbi.nih.gov

Nicotene Anonymous World Services
P.O. Box 591777
San Francisco, CA 94159-1777
1-415-750-0328
www.nicotine-anonymous.org

Phoenix House
164 West 74th Street
New York, NY 10023
1-800-HELP-111
www.acde.org

Substance Abuse and Mental Health Services Administration
5600 Fishers Lane
Rockville, MD 20857
1-800-662-HELP
1-800-WORKPLACE
www.samhsa.gov

Glossary

The glossary contains all keywords and their definitions. Keywords that are in capital letters are also entries. The volume(s) in which each keyword appears is indicated in brackets.

A

acupuncture an alternative treatment in which the healthcare provider inserts tiny needles at key places on the patient's body to relieve pain or other symptoms [Vols. 6, 8]

adrenaline hormone that stimulates the heart and other organs to prepare for fighting or fleeing from danger [Vol. 2]

aerobics physical activity that increases the flow of oxygen to the body [Vol. 3]

afterbirth the placenta and associated membranes that are expelled after delivery of an infant [Vol. 3]

agoraphobia a strong and irrational fear of open or public spaces; agoraphobics typically choose to remain in their own homes, only leaving if they can be escorted by someone they trust [Vol. 2]

allergens common everyday substances to which the body's immune system is oversensitive [Vol. 8]

ambient existing or present on all sides [Vol. 6]

amnesia a complete or partial loss of memory [Vol. 2]

ANABOLIC STEROIDS a group of steroids that are similar to the male hormone testosterone, which gives most men larger bodies and bigger skeletal muscles than the typical woman [Vol. 4]

anesthetic drug that produces anesthesia, an insensitivity to pain and other sensations [Vol. 1]

angina chest pains that occur as the result of coronary artery disease, which slows blood flow to the heart muscle [Vol. 4]

ANTIBIOTICS agents that fight bacteria [Vol. 8]

antibodies substances made by the body to attack foreign organisms or chemicals [Vols. 3, 8]

antigens foreign organisms that can provoke an immune response from the body [Vol. 8]

anti-inflammatory an agent that reduces the swelling, pain, redness, and heat usually associated with injury [Vol. 3]

antioxidants a type of phytochemical that seems to prevent cell damage from oxidation, or the loss of electrons, caused by the actions of free radicals; vitamins C and E are antioxidants [Vol. 4]

antiretroviral drug drug used to treat retroviruses, particularly HIV [Vol. 7]

appestat the part of the brain that controls eating behavior [Vol. 4]

appetite suppressants drugs taken to decrease the sense of hunger [Vol. 4]

aquifers underground pools that collect, store, and transfer groundwater [Vol. 6]

arson the deliberate act of starting a fire that destroys property [Vol. 5]

artificial sweeteners chemicals that imitate the sweetness of sugar but have fewer calories; they are used by people who suffer from diabetes mellitus or are trying to lose weight [Vol. 4]

aspartame one of the most popular artificial sweeteners in America; it is found in cereals, soft drinks, gum, yogurt, and low-calorie dessert foods [Vol. 4]

ATHEROSCLEROSIS narrowing of coronary arteries due to a buildup of deposits in them [Vol. 8]

B

bacteria microscopic, one-celled organisms that live both inside and outside the body, some of which can cause disease [Vols. 7, 8]

barrier methods contraceptive methods such as the condom, female condom, and cervical cap or diaphragm that create physical barriers between the sperm and the ovum [Vol. 3]

behavior therapy form of psychotherapy that uses learning and conditioning techniques to change undesirable behavior [Vol. 1]

benign pertaining to noncancerous cells not likely to grow or spread out of control [Vol. 8]

beriberi a disease that occurs when a person does not have enough vitamin B-1, or thiamine, and feels too sick to do anything; the legs become stiff, paralyzed, and painful [Vol. 4]

BIRTH DEFECTS abnormalities present before or after birth [Vol. 3]

blastocyst the embryonic stage at which the fertilized cell implants itself in the uterine wall [Vol. 3]

BLOOD ALCOHOL CONCENTRATION (BAC) the ratio of alcohol volume to blood volume in the body, expressed as a percent [Vols. 1, 5]

blood volume the quantity of blood within the body [Vol. 3]

bone marrow the soft tissue that fills the cavities of most bones, where red blood cells are manufactured [Vol. 3]

C

caesarian the surgical delivery of a baby [Vol. 3]

caffeine a natural stimulant found in the plants used to make tea, coffee, chocolate; an additive found in many foods, including soft drinks and medications [Vol. 4]

capital punishment the legal killing of a person convicted of a crime [Vol. 5]

CARCINOGENS cancer-causing agents [Vol. 8]

carnotite a radioactive mineral that is the source of uranium [Vol. 6]

cell division the means by which cells develop [Vol. 3]

cervix the narrow opening to the uterus [Vol. 3]

CHILD ABUSE physical harm to a child; sexual abuse of a child entails sexual gratification of an adult [Vol. 1]

child neglect failure to provide food, shelter, and medical attention; abandonment is a form of child neglect [Vol. 1]

CHOLESTEROL fatlike substance manufactured by the body and found in certain foods [Vol. 8]

chromosomes threadlike bodies in the nucleus of living cells that carry genes [Vol. 1]

circulatory system the body system through which blood flows [Vol. 3]

CMV retinitis an eye disease caused by cytomegalovirus (CMV) that often occurs in patients with AIDS [Vol. 7]

coma a state of deep, often prolonged unconsciousness, usually the result of injury, disease, or poison, in which a person does not respond to internal or external demands [Vol. 5]

compulsions repeated ritualized behaviors [Vol. 2]

contraception voluntary prevention of pregnancy [Vol. 3]

contraceptive methods chemical, physical, or hormonal methods used to prevent pregancy [Vol. 3]

contractions the pushing action of the uterus during labor [Vol. 3]

controlled substance drugs or other agents that are highly controlled and monitored by the Drug Enforcement Adminstration (DEA) [Vol. 2]

corrosive a substance that gradually weakens or destroys its surroundings such as a chemical that is capable of destroying the metal tank in which it is contained [Vol. 6]

craving intensely urgent need for an addictive substance such as alcohol, tobacco, or illegal drugs [Vol. 1]

crowning the first emergence of the fetus outside the birth canal [Vol. 3]

D

DATE RAPE DRUGS tasteless and odorless drugs that, when added to alcohol, often lead to unconsciousness and difficulty in remembering and that are favored by those who take sexual advantage of others [Vol. 5]

decibel a unit used to measure the relative intensity of sound; abbreviated dB [Vol. 6]

delivery the birthing process [Vol. 3]

delusions false beliefs [Vol. 2]

denial refusing to see a difficult situation as it really is [Vol. 2]

depersonalization uncomfortable feeling of being unreal or detached from one's body or surroundings [Vol. 2]

desertification the spread of an arid environment into areas that were not previously desert [Vol. 6]

detection discovery, usually through testing, of a disease [Vol. 8]

DETOXIFICATION withdrawal of an addictive substance under close medical supervision [Vol. 2]

DIAPHRAGM a muscle in the chest that helps with breathing [Vol. 3]

dietician a person qualified to plan diets for people with special health concerns or for hospitals, schools, or nursing homes [Vol. 4]

dilation and evacuation (D&E) a procedure in which the cervix is opened and the contents of the uterous are removed [Vol. 3]

dilation and extraction (D&X) a procedure in which the cervix is opened and the fetus is removed [Vol. 3]

disenfranchised describes individuals who have little or no power to influence social or political policies that affect them directly [Vol. 5]

disorientation loss of the sense of time or place [Vol. 2]

dissociation mentally separating oneself from a stressful event [Vol. 2]

diuretic substance that increases the volume of urine excreted from the kidneys [Vols. 1, 4]

domestic partner a person who lives with another [Vol. 5]

dopamine chemical in the brain that helps transmit messages between brain cells [Vol. 2]

dysthymia a mild form of depression that lasts for at least two years [Vol. 2]

E

eclampsia a general seizure that may be experienced by a woman after the 24th week of pregnancy [Vol. 3]

effluent waste matter discharged into the environment [Vol. 6]

electroconvulsive therapy treatment in which an electric current is passed through the brain of the anesthetized patient [Vol. 2]

electromagnetic radiation the transfer of energy produced by the motion of electrically charged particles [Vol. 6]

electromagnetic spectrum the range of electromagnetic waves, from the shortest to the longest [Vol. 6]

emission something that is released or discharged [Vol. 6]

endometrium the outer lining of the uterine wall [Vol. 3]

endorphins and enkephalins natural substances produced by the brain to reduce pain; these chemicals are also released during strenuous exercise, such as marathon racing [Vol. 4]

endurance the ability of the body to withstand physical stress or repetition [Vol. 4]

euphoria an exaggerated feeling of well-being that has no basis in reality [Vol. 1]

euthanasia enabling or assisting a person with terminal or painful illness to die [Vol. 5]

F

fertile able to conceive [Vol. 3]

fetal death the death of a fetus after week 28 of a pregnancy [Vol. 3]

flashback unexpected recurrence of the effects of a hallucinogenic drug long after its original use [Vol. 1]

foreskin a retractable fold of skin over the head of the penis [Vol. 3]

free radicals molecules having at least one unpaired electron that appear to cause certain diseases and to be involved in the aging process [Vol. 4]

frequency the number of waves that pass a certain point during one second [Vol. 6]

fructose sugar found in fruits, saps, and some vegetables [Vol. 4]

fungi plantlike organisms, including molds and mushrooms; some fungi can cause infections [Vol. 8]

G

genes the part of living cells that carries specific characteristics and passes them on from one generation to the next [Vol. 1, 7]

gestation the time a fetus spends developing in the uterous, from conception to birth [Vol. 3]

glucose a sugar that is the main fuel for body cells [Vol. 8]

goiter a condition in which the thyroid gland becomes swollen; one cause is too little iodine in the diet [Vol. 4]

glycogen a starch stored in the muscles that can be converted into glucose for energy [Vol. 4]

graffiti markings, initials, and sketches on walls, fences, and sidewalks, often used by gangs to mark territories [Vol. 5]

H

HALLUCINATIONS false perceptions [Vol. 2]

hate speech public communication that expresses the speaker's hatred, disapproval, or prejudice against certain groups of people [Vol. 5]

HEART ATTACK damage or even death to a part of the heart muscle that occurs when blood flow to the area is stopped because of a blood clot or coronary artery disease [Vols. 4, 8]

hernia a protrusion of an organ or tissue through an opening in its surrounding walls especially in the abdominal region of the body [Vol. 1]

heterosexism prejudice or discrimination against homosexuals [Vol. 5]

highly active antiretroviral therapy (HAART) a combination of several—usually three—antiretroviral drugs used to treat HIV and AIDS; often called an "AIDS cocktail" [Vol. 7]

homeopathy treatment of a disease in which small doses of a remedy that in a healthy person would produce symptoms of the disease being treated [Vols. 6, 8]

HORMONES chemical substances produced by glands that affect the functions of body organs and tissues [Vols. 1, 4]

hydrocarbons compounds containing carbon and hydrogen [Vol. 6]

hymen a thin membrane that partly covers the vagina, which may be torn by sexual intercourse [Vol. 3]

hyperbaric treatment placing a serverely burned patient in a chamber in which air pressure is raised to expose burns to high levels of oxygen for faster healing [Vol. 5]

I

implantation the positioning of a blastocyst in the uterine wall [Vol. 3]

INSULIN a hormone that enables cells to absorb glucose [Vol. 8]

irritable bowel syndrome (IBS) a condition in which irregular muscular movements in the small intestine and colon cause constipation, gas, bloating, and severe pain [Vol. 4]

J

jaundice a disease caused by an accumulation of bodily waste products in the blood when liver function is impaired, which causes the skin and eyes to turn yellow [Vol. 7]

juveniles persons under the age of 18 [Vol. 5]

L

lactose sugar found in milk and other dairy products [Vol. 4]

lactose intolerance a condition in which the small intestine fails to produce the enzyme, lactase, which is needed to break down milk, sugar, or lactose; the result is gas, bloating, and diarrhea [Vol. 4]

laparoscopy surgical inspection of the abdominal cavity and pelvis through a lit tube [Vol. 3]

LIFE EXPECTANCY the number of years a person is expected to live [Vol. 5]

life support artificial means of sustaining life [Vol. 5]

ligaments bands of tough tissue that tie bones to one another to form joints [Vol. 4]

lymphocyte a type of white blood cell that helps the immune system fight off infection and disease [Vol. 7]

M

macrophage a large white blood cell that surrounds and destroys microbes and is part of the immune system [Vol. 7]

malignant pertaining to cancerous cells that are likely to spread uncontrollably and to damage tissues of the body; cancerous [Vol. 8]

malnutrition condition of poor or unhealthy nutrition brought on by an inadequate or unbalanced diet [Vol. 1]

metabolize break down chemically within the body [Vol. 1]

METASTASIS process of malignant tumor cells spreading beyond their starting point in the body [Vol. 8]

microbe germ [Vol. 7]

microbicides agents that kill viruses and bacteria [Vol. 7]

microorganisms extremely small organisms, primarily bacteria, fungi, protozoa, and viruses [Vol. 6]

mill tailings the waste removed from an underground mine, which includes small particles of mine waste as well as rocks and other unmarketable materials [Vol. 6]

MORTALITY death [Vol. 5]

mutation unregulated changes in cells [Vol. 8]

mutual masturbation sexual stimulation in which two people bring each other to orgasm, either at the same time or one after the other, without intercourse [Vol. 7]

N

naturopathy treatment of a disease that emphasizes the use of natural agents such as heat, cold, water, sunshine, and physical therapies [Vols. 6, 8]

negotiation process in which differences are worked out and a solution is reached [Vol. 5]

neurotransmitter a substance that carries signals from one nerve cell to another [Vol. 2]

neutrophil a large white blood cell containing small sacs filled with enzymes that digest and destroy microbes and is part of the immune system [Vol. 7]

nicotine a toxic and highly addictive drug found in tobacco [Vol. 1]

nitrates additives used in cured meats to protect against food poisoning; has been linked to the production of possible cancer-causing agents in the human stomach [Vol. 4]

nomadic roaming from place to place [Vol. 6]

Nonoxynol-9 the active ingredient in spermicides available in the United States, which kills the sperm or inhibits its movement [Vol. 3]

norephinephrine a hormone and a neurotransmitter that causes heart rate, blood pressure, and blood sugar levels to increase and the blood vessels to constrict, preparing the body to meet stressful challenges [Vol. 2]

nuclei the plural of *nucleus;* the positively charged center of an atom [Vol. 6]

nutrient a substance found in foods, drinks, or diet supplements that the body needs to be able to grow, heal from injuries and illnesses, and perform daily functions; the six major nutrients are carbohydrates, fats, proteins, water, vitamins, and minerals [Vol. 4]

nutritionist a person who studies how food affects health and well-being [Vol. 4]

O

obsessions recurring disturbing thoughts or mental images [Vol. 2]

opportunistic infections rare infections that occur in people with weakened immune systems [Vol. 7]

ORGASM the peak or climax of sexual stimulation; in men, the ejaculation of semen from the penis; in women, the rhythmic contraction of the muscles around the vagina [Vol. 7]

ostracized excluded from participation [Vol. 5]

overuse injury an injury caused by repetitive motion [Vol. 4]

ovulation the release of an ovum from the ovary [Vol. 3]

oxytocin the hormone that makes labor start [Vol. 3]

P

panic attack sudden feeling of terror accompanied by physical sensations of extreme fear [Vol. 2]

paralysis the inability to move muscles, such as those in the legs and arms [Vol. 5]

paranoia irrational belief that others are out to harm you, a feature of some mental illnesses [Vols. 1, 2, 5]

paraplegic person who is paralyzed from the waist down [Vol. 5]

parasite organism that lives in or on another organism called a host; parasites depend on hosts for all of their nourishment [Vols. 7, 8]

parasitosis hallucination that many insects are crawling over or under the skin [Vol. 1]

parole the release of a convicted criminal from prison under strict conditions [Vol. 5]

particulates very small, separate particles; can be liquid droplets or tiny solid particles [Vol. 6]

passive smoking breathing in secondhand smoke, or smoke that is generated by another person [Vol. 1]

pathogens organisms that cause disease [Vol. 8]

PEER PRESSURE influence exerted on a person by their friends and other contemporaries [Vol. 5]

pellagra a disease that involves weakness, lack of appetite, diarrhea, and indigestion; it develops from not having enough vitamin B-3 or niacin and the amino acid tryptophan in the diet [Vol. 4]

perineum the area surrounding the genital and excretory organs [Vol. 3]

phytochemicals substances found in some plant foods such as fresh fruits and vegetables that seem to help prevent diseases [Vol. 4]

pitchblende a brownish-black mineral that contains large amounts of uraninite [Vol. 6]

plateau the point in a weight-loss program at which a person finds it difficult to lose any more weight [Vol. 4]

point source pollutants contaminants from a known source such as a drainage pipe [Vol. 6]

premature labor labor that occurs before the fetus is fully developed and ready to be born and survive on its own, usually defined as before week 38 of pregnancy [Vol. 3]

productivity ability to get things done and produce results; the rate of production [Vol. 6]

primary standards standards set by the Clean Air Act to protect public health [Vol. 6]

psychoactive capable of causing dramatic mood changes [Vol. 1]

purging trying to counteract overeating by vomiting, using laxatives, enemas, diuretics, or excessive exercise or dieting [Vol. 4]

R

racism prejudice or discrimination based on race or ethnicity [Vol. 5]

relapse a return to using an addictive substance after attempting to give it up [Vol. 1]

repression the burying of a painful memory or emotion [Vol. 2]

resistance the ability of a body to develop immunity to certain foods, drugs, toxins, diseases, or other stimuli [Vol. 7]

resuscitated brought back to life by forcing the heart to pump and blowing air into the lungs; also called cardiopulmonary resuscitation, or CPR [Vol. 3]

RETROVIRUS virus that infects cells by inserting its RNA into them, instead of DNA as most viruses do [Vol. 7]

R.I.C.E the usual treatment for sprains: rest, ice, compress, and elevate [Vol. 4]

rickets childhood bone disease often caused by a lack of calcium, phosphate, or vitamin D; the bones become soft, bent, bumpy, and abnormally shaped [Vol. 4]

risk factors factors that increase someone's chances of getting a disease but do not necessarily cause it [Vol. 8]

rush a sudden feeling of intense euphoria brought on by the use of certain drugs [Vol. 1]

S

safe houses places where victims of domestic abuse can live temporarily free of abuse and harassment [Vol. 5]

satiety the sense of fullness that comes at the end of a meal [Vol. 4]

secondary standards set by the Clean Air Act to protect public welfare [Vol. 6]

SELF-HELP GROUPS collections of people with similar problems or in similar situations who come together for aid and support [Vol. 5]

serotonin a hormone and a neurotransmitter that helps transmit messages between cells, stimulate smooth muscles, and regulate learning, sleep, and mood; found in the brain, blood, serum, and the mucous membrane of the stomach [Vol. 2]

sexism prejuicice or discrimination based on sex [Vols. 3, 5]

side-stream smoke the smoke that a nonsmoker inhales from the environment [Vol. 1]

sludge in sewage treatment, thick, solid matter that has settled out of wastewater in tanks or basins [Vol. 6]

SOBRIETY CHECKPOINTS roadblocks set up to stop, identify, and arrest those who are driving while intoxicated [Vol. 5]

social norms behaviors generally expected and accepted by society [Vol. 5]

social pressures influences in society to think, choose, or act in certain ways [Vol. 5]

socioeconomic status the position a person or group has in society based on family background, education, and income [Vol. 5]

speculum a long, hollow, lighted device used to view the inside of the vagina and cervix [Vol. 3]

stalking following or pursuing another person in a menacing way or with apparent intent to injure them [Vol. 5]

starch complex carbohydrates found in foods such as breads, cereals, pastas, and rice; some vegetables, especially corn and potatoes, also contain a lot of starch; during digestion starches are broken down into simple sugars, which are used as a fuel for body activities [Vol. 4]

sterile unable to produce or support life; unproductive [Vol. 6]

stillbirth a baby that is born dead [Vol. 3]

substance abuse excessive use of alcohol, drugs, tobacco, or other addictive substances [Vol. 1]

sucrose table sugar; processed from sugarcane and sugar beet plants and used as a sweetener [Vol. 4]

sulfites preservatives found in a range of products, including potato chips, bottled juices, and canned fruits, vegetables, and soups; can cause allergic reactions, including asthma attacks [Vol. 4]

T

tendon a band or cord of tissue that connects a muscle to a bone [Vol. 4]

teratogens substances such as cigarette smoke, alcohol, and some drugs, which are known to cause birth defects [Vols. 1, 3]

tinnitus a constant ringing in the ears caused by damage to the auditory nerve [Vol. 6]

TOLERANCE capacity of the body to endure or become less responsive to a substance with repeated use [Vols. 1, 2]

transfusion the transfer of one person's blood into another person's body [Vol. 7]

transuranic wastes wastes created from the production of nuclear fuel and weapons, such as protective clothing, equipment, tools, and contaminated soils [Vol. 6]

tremors trembling or shaking [Vol. 2]

TUMOR mass of cells produced as a result of uncontrolled cellular growth [Vol. 8]

U

urethra tube that drains urine from the bladder to the outside of the body [Vol. 3]

uterine lining the buildup of blood and nutrients on the inside wall of the uterus that supports and protects the developing fetus [Vol. 3]

V

vegan a type of vegetarian who only eats plant-derived foods, excluding even animal by-products, such as eggs, milk, and butter [Vol. 6]

VIRUSES infectious microorganisms that can enter the body, target particular types of tissues, and damage cells [Vols. 7, 8]

volatile organic compounds substances that react with sunlight to form new pollutant compounds [Vol. 6]

Z

zygote a fertilized ovum [Vol. 3]

Further Reading and Internet Sites

For Volume 1: *Addiction: Tobacco, Alcohol, and Other Drugs*

Braun, Stephen. *Buzz: The Science and Lore of Alcohol and Caffeine*. New York: Penguin USA, 1997.

Friedman, Lawrence, Nicholas F. Fleming, David H. Roberts, and Steven E. Hyman, eds. *Source Book of Substance Abuse and Addiction*. Baltimore: Williams & Wilkins, 1996.

Jonnes, Jill. *Hep Cats, Narcs, and Pipe Dreams: A History of America's Romance with Illegal Drugs*. New York: Simon & Schuster, 1996.

Knapp, Caroline. *Drinking: A Love Story*. New York: Dell Publishing Company, 1997.

Kuhn, Cynthia. *Buzzed: The Straight Facts about the Most Used and Abused Drugs from Alcohol to Ecstasy*. New York: W.W. Norton, 1998.

Levenkron, Steven. *Obsessive-Compulsive Disorders: Treating and Understanding Crippling Habits*. New York: Warner Books, 1992.

Maximin, Anita, and Lori Stevic-Rust. *The Stop Smoking Workbook*. New York: Fine Communications, 1997.

McCoy, Kathy, and Charles Wibbelsman. *Life Happens: A Teenager's Guide to Friends, Failure, Sexuality, Love, Rejection, Addiction, Peer Pressure, Families, Loss, Depression, Change, and Other Challenges of Living*. New York: Berkeley Publishing Group, 1996.

McGovern, George. *Terry: My Daughter's Life and Death Struggle with Alcoholism*. New York: Dutton, 1997.

Sandmaier, Marian. *The Invisible Alcoholics: Women and Alcohol*. New York: TAB Books, 1997.

Schuckit, Marc Alan. *Educating Yourself about Alcohol and Drugs: A Peoples' Primer*. New York: Plenum, 1998.

Scott, Tom, and Trevor Grice. *The Great Brain Robbery*. Green Bay, WI: Recovery Works Publishing, 1997.

Weil, Andrew, and Winifred Rosen. *From Chocolate to Morphine: Everything You Need to Know about Mind-Altering Drugs*. Boston: Houghton Mifflin, 1993.

Wurtzel, Elizabeth. *Prozac Nation: Young and Depressed in America*. New York: Berkeley Publishing Group, 1997.

Zimmer, Lynn and John P. Morgan. *Marijuana Myths, Marijuana Facts: A Review of the Scientific Evidence*. New York: Open Society Institute, 1997.

http://tobaccofreekids.org [Campaign for Tobacco-Free Kids] *Looks critically at the public relations and advertising campaigns of tobacco companies and presents current research on the effects of smoking.*

http://people.delphi.com/mickjyoung/drugs.html [Mickey's Drug and Drug Abuse Prevention Resources] *Provides a comprehensive collection of resources with annotations, including clearinghouses, directories, crime, and more.*

www.ndsn.org [National Drug Strategy Network] *Offers information on drug-related problems and prevention, including news briefs, law enforcement, policy reform, treatment help, government agencies, prevention centers, civil liberties, crime data, and sentencing.*

www.inhalants.com [National Inhalant Prevention Coalition] *About inhalants and how to recognize who is using them; includes statistics and prevention resources.*

www.well.com/user/woa/woarollo.htm [Web of Addictions] *Provides an excellent list of hotlines, help numbers, and support groups for alcohol and drug addictions.*

For the Set

American Academy of Family Physicians. *Family Health and Medical Guide.* Dallas: Word Publishing, 1996.

American College of Physicians. *American College of Physicians Complete Home Medical Guide.* New York: DK Publishing, 1999.

American Medical Association. *American Medical Association Family Medical Guide.* New York: Random House, 1994.

American Medical Women's Association. *The Women's Complete Healthbook.* New York: Dell Publishing Company, Inc., 1997.

Anderson, Kenneth N., ed. *Mosby's Medical Dictionary.* St. Louis: Mosby, 1994.

Barrett, Stephen, et al. *Consumer Health.* New York: McGraw-Hill, 1997.

Berkow, Robert, and Mark H. Beers, eds. *The Merck Manual of Medical Information: Home Edition.* Whitehouse Station, NJ: Merck Research Laboratories, 2000.

Caravella, Philip. *The Art of Being a Patient: Taming Medicine: An Insider's Guide: Become a Proactive Partner and Self-Advocate of Your Own Health by Understanding.* Bloomington, IN: 1st Books Library, 2000.

Columbia University College of Physicians and Surgeons. *The Columbia University College of Physicians and Surgeons Complete Home Medical Guide.* New York: Crown, 1995.

Columbia University's Health Education Program. *The Go Ask Alice Book of Answers: A Guide to Good Physical, Sexual, and Emotional Health.* New York: Henry Holt, 1998.

Eniola, Anthony. *ABCs of Healthy Living.* Hallandale, FL: Aglob Publishing, 2001.

Faber, Adele, and Elaine Mazlish. *How to Talk So Kids Will Listen & How to Listen So Kids Will Talk.* Mamaroneck, NY: International Center for Creative Thinking, 1990.

Harvard Medical School. *Harvard Medical School Family Health Guide.* New York: Simon & Schuster, 1999.

Mayo Clinic. *Mayo Clinic Family Health Book: The Ultimate Home Reference.* New York: William Morrow, 1998.

Tipley, Donald F., Thomas Q. Morris, and Lewis P. Rowland. *The Columbia University College of Physicians and Surgeons Complete Home Medical Guide.* New York: Crown, 1985.

www.healthatoz.com [Health A to Z: Your Family Health Site]
Offers interactive tools for setting up a personal health calendar, homepage, prescription reminders, and subscriptions to health news; offers opportunities to e-mail healthcare professionals and chat with users.

www.healthfinder.com [Healthfinder]
Gives teens advice on prevention, self-care, and quality care; offers access to health-related library services, news, and professional research; run by the U.S. Department of Health and Human Services.

www.mayoclinic.com [Mayo Clinic]
Offers interactive tools to help you "take charge of your health," including a personal health scorecard, healthy lifestyle planners, and decision guides; provides information on health topics and answers to frequently asked questions from Mayo specialists.

www.medicinenet.com [Medicine Net]
Provides consumer medical information from U.S. board-certified physicians, including guides to over-the-counter and prescription drugs.

www.reutershealth.com [Reuters Health]
Features links to consumer, industry, and professional health news.

www.nlm.nih.gov [United States National Library of Medicine]
Provides online catalog access to the world's largest medical library; features three databases: Medline Plus answers health questions, Medline/PubMed summarizes articles from medical journals, and Clinical Trials let you know about research studies.

Set Index

Bold numbers refer to volume numbers and page numbers of main entries. Page numbers in regular type indicate other mentions of entries and terms. *Italic* numbers and letters refer to charts *(c)*, marginal features *(f)*, illustrations *(i)*, and tables *(t)*.

A

AA (Alcoholics Anonymous), **1:48**, *149–150t*
abortion, **3:19–22**, *20c, 21i*
  choices and actions, 3:142
  late-term, *3:23f*
  laws concerning, 3:23–24
  risks from, 3:147
abstinence, 1:19, **3:24**, *24f*, 7:17–18
abuse, **5:19–20**
abuse and mental health, **2:19–20**
acceptance therapy, *2:60f*
accidents, **5:20–21**. *See also* injuries
acetaminophen, *1:118f*
acid. *See* LSD
acid rain, **6:14–15**, *16i*, 78–79
ACTH, 7:18
activity and nutrition, **4:21–22**
acupuncture, 6:20, 8:26
addiction, **1:20–21**, **8:21–22**, *22t*
  alcohol, **1:36–38**
  causes of, 1:23
  cost of, *1:21f*
  deaths from, **1:71–73**, *71f*
  to food, 4:61
  genetics and, 1:23–24
  injuries and, 1:24–25
  medications for, **1:25–26**
  mental health and, **2:20–22**, *22c*
  peer pressure and, **1:121**
  prescription drugs and, **1:21–23**, 158
  signs of, 1:26–27
  to smoking, 1:166–167
  to smoking, quitting, **1:128–130**, 167–168
  stages of, 1:26–27
  teens and, *1:134c*, 135–136, *136t*
  tobacco, **1:137–140**
  withdrawal, 1:150
addiction, causes of, **1:23**
addiction, genetics and, **1:23–24**
addiction, injuries and, **1:24–25**
addiction, medications for, **1:25–26**
addiction, signs of, **1:26–27**
addiction, stages of, **1:26–27**
additives in food, **4:22–23**
ADHD. *See* attention deficit hyperactivity disorder
adipose tissue, **4:23**
adjustment disorder, **2:22–23**
adrenaline, 2:31, 70–71
advertising and media, **1:27–28**, **4:23–28**
aerobic exercise, 3:49, **4:28–29**
afterbirth, 3:90
agoraphobia, 2:70
agricultural pollution, **6:67–68**
  fertilizers and, **6:39–40**
AIDS, 1:103, **7:18–23**, *19f, 21f*, 8:22–23. *See also* HIV/AIDS
  confidentiality and, 7:37–38
  death and, 1:40–42
  mental health and, 2:23–24
  death and, **1:40–42**
  nutrition and, 7:23
  teens and, **7:100–101**, *100t*
  worldwide, 7:23–25, *24t*
AIDS and nutrition, **7:23**
AIDS in the world, **7:23–25**
AIDS and mental health, **2:23–24**
air bags, 5:21, *21f*
airborne transmission of infections. *See* infectious diseases
air pollution, **6:16–17**, *17t, 29i*
air quality, **6:17–19**
  concerns and fears, 6:92–93
  emission trends of pollutants, *6:19c*
  miners and, 6:55–56
  pollutant standards index, 6:66–67, *66c*
Al-Anon, **1:30–31**
Alateen, **1:31**
alcohol, **1:31–32**. *See also* alcohol abuse; alcohol addiction; alcoholism, alcohol use addiction. *See* alcohol addiction
  blackouts, 1:47–48
  cocaine and, *1:67f*
  dependence in U.S., *1:37t*
  depression and, 2:122–123
  drug/medication interactions with, 1:45–47, *46t*
  drugs and sex and, 1:41–42, 7:25–26
  effects, 1:31–32
  experimentation, 1:47
  health problems and, **1:42–45**, *43f*
  injuries and, 5:21–22
  laws regulating, 1:51–52, *52c*
  mental health and, 2:24–25, *25t–26t*
  metabolism of, 1:52
  overdose, 1:53, 5:22–23
  poisoning, 1:53–54
  pregnancy and, 3:24–25
  risks of injury from, 1:153–155
  sex and. *See* sex, alcohol, and drugs
  violence and, 1:45, 5:22
  weight and, 4:29–30
alcohol abuse, **1:32–36**
  behavior problems due to, 1:161–162
  child abuse and, 1:65–66
  health risks from, 1:13–15
  health risks to women, 1:155–156. *See also* alcohol
alcohol addiction, **1:36–38**, *37i. See also* alcohol
  counseling, 1:38–39
  rehabilitation programs, **1:39–40**
alcohol, causes of, **1:36–38**
alcohol, drugs and sex and, 1:41–42, **3:115–116**, *115f*, 7:25–26
alcoholic psychosis, **8:23–24**
Alcoholics Anonymous (AA), **1:48**, *149–150t*
alcoholism, **1:49**, 8:24. *See also* addiction, alcohol
  risks of developing, 1:169–170
  treatment of, **1:49–81**, *8:24t*
alcohol use, **1:30**. *See also* alcohol
  in college, 1:77–79
  eating and caffeine and, 1:170
  falling down and, 1:154–155
  fetal alcohol syndrome, 1:96–97
  health risks from, 1:10
  malnutrition and, 1:40–41
  mood and, 1:41
  during pregnancy, 1:123
  sex and, 1:41–42
allergens, **8:25**
allergies, 6:23, **8:25**. *See also* asthma
  to food, 4:61–62
alternative medicine, **1:54–56**, **2:27–29**, *27f*, **3:25–27**, **4:30–31**, **5:23–25**, **6:20**, **7:26–27**, **8:25–27**
Alzheimer's disease, **8:27**
amino acids, **4:31–32**
amnesia, 1:120, 2:45
amphetamines, **1:56–57**
amyl nitrate, **1:57–58**
amyotrophic lateral sclerosis (ALS), **8:28**
anabolic steroids, **1:58**, 91–92, 4:114
anaerobic exercise, **4:32**
anal intercourse/anal sex, **3:27–28**, 7:27–28
androgens, **3:28**
androgyny, **3:28**
anemia, **4:32–33**, 8:28–29
anesthetic, 1:67, 120
aneurysm, **8:29**
angel dust, **1:120**
angina pectoris, 4:45, **8:29**
angioplasty, **8:29–30**
annual exam, **3:28–29**

anorexia nervosa, **2**:51, **4**:33–34. *See also* eating disorders

antabuse, **1**:58

anterior cruciate ligament (ACL), **4**:139–140

antibiotics, **1**:58–59, **7**:28, **8**:30, *30f, 99f*

antibodies, **1**:125, **3**:*65f*, **8**:25, *99f*

antidepressants, **2**:29–30, *30i*

antigens, **8**:*99f*

anti-inflammatory, **3**:78

antioxidants, **4**:102

antiretroviral drugs, **7**:40, 93

antismoking laws, **1**:59

antismoking products, **1**:59–61

anxiety, **2**:30–31, *31i*

aphrodisiac, **3**:29

appendicitis, **8**:30–31

appestat, **4**:34

appetite and hunger, **4**:34–35

appetite suppressants, **4**:34

aquifers, **6**:*85f*

arrhythmia, **8**:31

arsenic, **6**:20–21

arson, **5**:68

arteriosclerosis, **8**:31

arthritis, **8**:31–32

artificial sweeteners, **4**:22

artificial wetlands, **6**:*76f*

asbestos, **6**:21–22, *21f*

asbestosis, **8**:32

aspartame, **4**:22

asphyxiation, **6**:22

assault, **5**:25

asthma, **1**:61, **6**:22–23, **8**:32–33

  exercise and, **4**:144–145

  atherosclerosis, **8**:33, 63

attention deficit hyperactivity disorder (ADHD), **2**:33–35, *33t, 35f,* 116–117

autoimmune disorders, **8**:33, **111**

automobile accidents. *See* motor-vehicle injuries

AZT, **7**:28–29

B

baby blues, **2**:*76f*, **3**:93

BAC (blood alcohol concentration), **1**:*53*, 63, *80t,* **5**:*49f, 50t*

back injuries, **5**:26

back pain, chronic, **8**:55–56

bacteria, **1**:138, **7**:23, **8**:25

bacterial infections, **8**:34

bacterial vaginosis, **3**:30

balanced diet. *See* nutrition, health and

barbiturates, **1**:61–62

barrier methods, **3**:*125f*

basal metabolic rate (BMR), **4**:35–36

bathtub drowning, **5**:46, 48

beer, **1**:62, *62f*

behavioral therapy, **1**:49, **2**:35–36

behavior problems and alcohol/drug abuse, **1**:158–159

benign tumors, **8**:36, 41

beriberi, **4**:*121f*

Bhopal, India gas leak, **6**:36, 96–97

bicycling, **4**:36

  helmet use, **8**:19, *77f*

  injuries, **5**:26–27, *92f*

  safety, **5**:27–28

bidis, **1**:*144f*

binge drinking, **1**:53–54, 62–63, *78t*

biochemical oxygen demand (BOD), **6**:76

biofeedback, **8**:25, 75

bipolar disorder, **2**:36–37, 68

birth-control implants, **3**:30–31

birth-control shot, **3**:31

birth defects, **3**:31–32

birth rates, unmarried women, **3**:*52c*

bisexuality, **7**:29–30

Black Death, **8**:101

black lung disease, **6**:24, **8**:34–35

blackouts from alcohol use, **1**:47–48

bladder cancer, **8**:35

blastocyst, **3**:*37f*

blindness, **8**:87, 140

blood alcohol concentration (BAC), **1**:53, 63, 80–81, *80t,* **5**:*49f, 50t*

blood alcohol levels, **1**:63

blood poisoning, **8**:35

blood pressure, **1**:102–103, **4**:67–88, 105, **8**:93–94, *94t,* 110

blood safety, **7**:30–31

blood sugar. *See* diabetes mellitus

blood volume, **3**:102

BMR (basal metabolic rate), **4**:35–36

body image, **4**:19–20, 36–37

body mass index (BMI), **4**:37–38

bone fractures, **4**:136–137

bone marrow, **3**:102

bone marrow transplants, **8**:35–36

Braille typewriters, **8**:*76i*

brain injuries, **5**:107–108

brain tumor, **8**:36–37

breast cancer, **8**:37–38, *37t*

breast self-exam, **3**:32

bronchitis, **1**:63–64, **8**:38

bubonic plague, **8**:125–126

bulimia nervosa, 19, **2**:51, *51f,* **4**:38–39, 140–142, **8**:9. *See also* eating disorders

bullying, **5**:28–29

burn injuries, **5**:29–33, *31f, 32t*

burns, chemical, **6**:24–25, 41–42

bursitis, **8**:38–39

bypass surgery, **8**:50

C

cadmium, **6**:*31f*

caffeine, **8**:*153t*

calorie, **4**:39–41, *40t*

cancer, **1**:64, **8**:41–47. *See also specific types*

  death rates, **8**:*42f, 42t*

  diets and, **4**:41

  exercise and, **4**:42

  metastasis, **8**:117

  number of new cases, **8**:*40c*

  testing for, **8**:39

  treatment of, **8**:47–48

  warning signs of, **8**:39–41

cancer, testing for, **8**:39

cancer treatments, **8**:47–48

cancer, warning signs of, **8**:39–41

candidiasis, **3**:33, **7**:32

cannabis. *See* hashish; marijuana

capital punishment, **5**:*77f*

car accidents. *See* motor-vehicle injuries

carbohydrates, **4**:42–43

carbon monoxide, **6**:26, *26f*

  health risks from, **6**:99

  laws regulating, **6**:52–53

  monitoring, **6**:26–27

  sources and effects, **6**:*17t*

carcinogens, **1**:65, **8**:41

  environmental, **6**:27

carcinoma, **8**:48–49

car crashes and teens, **1**:153–154. *See also* motor-vehicle injuries

cardiac arrest, **8**:*49t,* 49–50

cardiac rehabilitation, **4**:43–44

cardiopulmonary resuscitation (CPR), **8**:68

cardiorespiratory fitness rating, **4**:*96f, 97t*

cardiovascular disease, treatment of, **8**:50–51

cardiovascular disease, types of, **8**:51

cardiovascular fitness, **8**:51–52

car emissions, **6**:27–28

carnotite, **6**:84

car safety seats, **5**:34–35, *34c*

cataracts, **8**:*84t*

CAT scan, **8**:52

CDC. *See* Centers for Disease Control and Prevention

cell division, **3**:*37f*

cellular phones, **6**:*70f*

Centers for Disease Control and Prevention (CDC), **1**:65, **2**:37–38, **3**:33–34, **4**:44, **5**:35, **6**:28–29, **7**:33, **8**:52

cerebral hemorrhage, **8**:52, **139**

cerebral palsy, **8**:52–53

cervical cancer, **8**:53

cervical cap, **3**:34

cervix, **3**:52

cesarean, **3**:*34f*

CFCs (chlorofluorocarbons), **6**:32

chancre, **7**:33–34

chancroid, **7**:34

chemical burns, **6**:24–25, 41–42

chemical pollution, **6**:29–32

chemical spills, **6**:96–97

Chernobyl explosion, **6**:37, 95–96

chewing tobacco, **1**:127–128

chicken pox, **8**:53–55, *54i*

child abuse, **1**:65–66, **5**:35–37, *36c*

childbirth, **3**:34–35

childhood obesity, **4**:*85f,* 142–143

child neglect, **1**:65
children and nutrition, **4**:*86t*, 144
chlamydia, **3**:35–36, **7**:34–35, *101f, 103t. See also* sexually transmitted diseases (STDs)
  concerns and fears, **7**:111–112
  teen example, **7**:117–118
chlorofluorocarbons (CFCs), **6**:32
cholera, **8**:55
cholesterol, **8**:63
chromosomes, **1**:24
chronic back pain, **8**:55–56
chronic diseases, **8**:56–58, *56t*
  treatment of, **8**:58–59
chronic fatigue syndrome, **8**:59–60
chronic obstructive pulmonary disease (COPD), **8**:60, *60t*
chronic stress, **2**:110–111
cigarettes. *See* tobacco
cigars. *See* tobacco
circulatory system, **3**:*102f*
cirrhosis of the liver, **1**:*43f*, 66
CJD (Creutzfeldt-Jakob Disease), **8**:68
Clean Air Acts, **6**:33. *See also* air quality
Clean Water Acts, **6**:33–34, *88f. See also* water pollution
climate. *See* greenhouse effect
clinical depression, **2**:115–116
clitoris, **3**:36
club drugs, **1**:66–67. *See also* designer drugs
CMV (cytomegalovirus), **7**:39–40
CMV retinitis, **7**:94
cocaine, **1**:67–68, *67f, 68i*, **8**:*22t*
codependency, **1**:69
cognitive therapy, **2**:38
cohabitation, **3**:36–37
coitus. *See* sexual intercourse
coitus interruptus (withdrawal), **3**:100
colitis, **8**:60–61
colorectal cancer, **8**:61
coma, **5**:67
common cold, **8**:61, *61f*
communicable diseases, **8**:62–63

compulsions, **2**:32
conception, **3**:37
condom, **3**:37–38, 146–147, **7**:35–36
condom availability programs, **7**:36–37
confidentiality and AIDS, HIV, and STDs, **7**:37–38
congenital diseases. *See* genetic disorders
congenital heart defects, **8**:91–92
congestive heart failure, **8**:62
conjunctivitis, **8**:62, *84t*
  gonococcal, **7**:47–48
conservation, **6**:34
contagious diseases, **8**:62–63
contraception, **3**:30, *51f. See also* pregnancy, prevention of
  cervical cap, **3**:34
  condom, **3**:37–38, 146–147, **7**:35–36
  Depo-Provera, **3**:31
  emergency contraceptive pills, **3**:47
  methods, **3**:*20f, 101t*, 142
  Nonoxynol-9, **3**:125
  Norplant, **3**:30–31
contractions, **3**:*34f*
controlled substances, **1**:88, 118
cooling-down period, **4**:44–45
COPD (Creutzfeldt-Jakob Disease), **8**:68
coronary heart disease, **4**:45, **8**:51, 63–67, *63f*
corrosive, **6**:47
cotinine, **6**:*31f*
counseling for violence issues, **5**:37
CPR (cardiopulmonary resuscitation), **8**:68
crabs (pubic lice), **7**:38–39
crack cocaine, **1**:69–70
Creutzfeldt-Jakob Disease (CJD), **8**:68
crossing signals, lights, stop signs, **5**:38
cross-training, **4**:45–46
crowning, **3**:34
curfews, **5**:38
cystic fibrosis, **8**:68
cystitis. *See* bacterial infections; infectious diseases
cytomegalovirus (CMV), **7**:39–40

D
dares, **5**:38
date rape, **5**:39
date rape drugs, **1**:70–71, **3**:38–39, **5**:40
dating, **3**:39–40
dating abuse, **3**:40–41, *40f*, **5**:39–40
DEA (Drug Enforcement Administration), **1**:86–87
death:
  from addiction, **1**:*43f*, 71–73, *71f*
  from cancer, **1**:64, *141f*, **8**:41–47
  from guns, **5**:62–63
  from HIV, AIDS, and STDs, **7**:40–42, *41f*
  from homicide, **5**:*69f*
  from smoking, **1**:*137f*
  from suicide, **2**:*99t*
death, leading causes of, **5**:40–41, *41t–42t. See also* morbidity
decibel levels, **6**:57
defense mechanisms, **2**:38–39
degenerative disorders, nervous system, **8**:69–70
delirium tremens (DTs), **1**:73–74
delivery, **3**:34
delusions, **2**:49
dementia, **2**:39–40, **8**:70
dengue fever, **8**:70
denial, **2**:39
dental dam, **7**:43
dependence, **1**:74
depersonalization, **2**:45, 46
Depo-Provera (birth-control shot), **3**:31
depressants, **1**:74–76, *75t*, **2**:*47t*
depression, **2**:40–45, *40f*, 115–116, **8**:70–71, *70f*
  alcohol and tobacco use and, **2**:122–123
  chances of developing, **2**:16–18
  smoking and, **5**:*105f*
  warning signs, **2**:119–120
desertification, **6**:35–36
designer drugs, **1**:76, *76f. See also* club drugs
detoxification, **1**:76–77, **2**:*21f*
diabetes mellitus, **4**:46–47, **8**:71–72
  gestational, **3**:56–57, **4**:67

diaphragm, **3**:41, 103
diet. *See also* nutrition; nutritional guidelines; nutritional planning
diet and pregnancy. *See* nutrition, pregnancy and
dietary supplements, **4**:47–48, **8**:*121f*
diet fads, **4**:48–49
dietician, **4**:77
digestion, **4**:49–50
dilation and evacuation (D&E), **3**:20, 22
dilation and extraction (D&X), **3**:20, 22
diptheria, **8**:75
disability, **2**:*67t*
disabling conditions, **8**:76–77
disabling conditions, treatment of, **8**:77
disasters, environmental, **6**:35–37, *35f, 36i*
disenfranchised, **5**:42
disorientation, **2**:*23f*
dissociation, **2**:39
dissociative disorders, **2**:45–46
diuretic, **1**:52, **4**:38
diverticulitis, **8**:77–78
diving injuries. *See* drowning
divorce, **3**:*76f*
domestic partner, **5**:42, 101
domestic violence:
  abuse and, **1**:77, **5**:41–44, *43f. See also* intimate partner violence
  shelters, **5**:44
donor cards, **8**:78
dopamine, **1**:113, **2**:80
douching, **3**:41–42
doula, **3**:42
Down syndrome, **8**:78
drinking in college, **1**:77–79
drive-by shootings, **5**:44–45
driving while intoxicated or drug impaired, **1**:80–82
drowning, **5**:45–48, *45t, 48f*
drowning sites, **5**:46, 48
drug abuse, **1**:82–86, *84t*, **8**:*22t*
  addiction and. *See* drug addiction
  child abuse and, **1**:65–66
  IV drug use, **7**:114
  malnutrition and, **1**:40–41
  mental health and, **2**:46–49, *47t, 48c*
  mood and, **1**:41

drug abuse (*Continued*)
  during pregnancy, **1:**123
  risks from, **1:**13–15
  STDs and, **7:**89–90
  substance abuse in U.S.,
    1:*84t*
  victims of, **1:***82f*
drug addiction, **1:**86
  counseling, **1:**38–39
  rehabilitation programs,
    1:39–40
Drug Enforcement
  Administration (DEA),
  1:86–87
drug-free zones, **1:**87
drug interactions, **1:**87
drug/medication interac-
  tions with alcohol,
  1:45–47, *46t*
drug possession, **1:**163
drugs, **1:**89–90, 154. *See
  also* illegal drugs;
  specific types
  alcohol and, **7:**25–26
  date rape and, **1:**70–71,
    3:38–39, **5:***38f*
  health problems and,
    1:90–93
  laws regulating, **1:**87–88
  mixing with prescription
    drugs, **1:**164–165
  overdose from, **1:**88–89,
    164–165, **5:**48–49
  pregnancy and,
    1:122–123, *122c*,
    3:43–44
  testing for, **1:**93–94
  treatment programs,
    7:43–44
drug therapy, **2:**49–50
drug treatment programs,
  7:43–44
drunk driving, **1:**51, *52c*,
  153–154, **5:**49–51, *51f*
drunk-driving laws, **5:**51
DTs (delirium tremens),
  1:73–74
DWI roadblocks, **5:**51–52
dysentery, **8:**78–79
dysthymia, **2:**44, 110

E

ear problems, **8:**78–79
eating disorders, **2:**50–52,
  51f, **4:**33–34, 50–51,
  140–142
eating out and nutrition,
  4:*76f*
Ebola hemorrhagic fever,
  8:80
eclampsia, **3:***65f*

ECPs (emergency contra-
  ceptive pills), **3:**47
ecstasy, **1:**94–95, *94f*
ectopic pregnancy,
  3:44–45, *45f*
effluent, **6:**30
egg. *See* ovum
ejaculation, **3:**45–46
elder abuse, **5:**52
electric-shock injuries. *See*
  burn injuries
electrocardiogram (ECG,
  EKG), **8:**80
electroconvulsive therapy,
  2:44
electromagnetic radiation,
  6:69
electromagnetic spectrum,
  6:70–71
embryo, **3:**46–47
emergencies and reporting
  environmental threats,
  6:35
emergency contraceptive
  pills (ECPs), **3:**47
emergency medical services
  (EMS), **5:**52–53
emergency response, **5:**53
emergency room treatment,
  5:53–54
emission, **6:**16
emotionally disturbed state.
  See mental illness
emphysema, **1:**95, **8:**81
empty calories, **4:**51–52
encephalitis, **8:**81
endocarditis, **8:**81–82
endometrium, **3:***110f*
endorphins, **4:**94
endurance, **4:**94
engagement, **3:**47–48
environmental disasters,
  6:35–37, 95–97
Environmental Protection
  Agency (EPA), **6:**37–38
ephedra, **8:**121
epidemiology, **1:**95–96,
  2:51–52, **3:**48, **4:**52, **5:**54,
  6:38, **7:**44–45, **8:**82
epilepsy, **8:**82–83
erectile dysfunction, **8:**83
erogenous zones, **3:**48–49
estrogen, **3:**49
euthanasia, **5:**101
exercise. *See also* physical
  activity and health
  flexibility and, **4:**52–53
  heat and sun exposure
    and, **4:**53–54, *54t*
  injuries and, **4:**54–56
  pregnancy and, **3:**49–50,
    50f, **4:**56

  strength and, **4:**56–57, *57f*
  weight and dieting and,
    4:57–58
exercise and flexibility,
  4:52–53
exercise and heat and sun
  exposure, **4:**53–54, *54t*
exercise-induced asthma,
  4:144–145
exercise and injuries,
  4:54–56
exercise and pregnacy,
  3:49–50, *50f*, **4:**56
exercise and strength,
  4:56–57, *57f*
exercise, weight, and, dieting, **4:**57–58
exposure guidelines, **6:**38–39
Exxon Valdez, **6:***61f*
eye disorders, **8:**83–84, *84t*

F

fad diets, **4:**48–49
falls and injuries, **5:**54–56
  alcohol use and,
    1:154–155
family, **3:**50–51
family abuse and mental
  health. *See* abuse and
  mental health
family planning, **3:**51–52
family therapy, **2:**52
family violence. *See* domestic violence, abuse and
fast foods, **4:**58–59
fatigue syndrome, chronic,
  8:59–60
fats, **4:**59–60
female condom, **3:**52–53
female sex organs,
  3:110–111
fertile, **3:**30
fertility awareness, **3:**53–54
fertility rates, **3:***54c*
fertilization, **3:**54–55
fertilizers, **6:**39–40, 99–100
fetal alcohol syndrome
  (FAS), **1:**96–97, 156
fetal death, **3:**103
fetus, **3:**55
fiber, **4:**60
fires:
  burn injuries, **5:**29–33,
    31f, 32t
  escape drills, **5:**56–57
  escape plans, **5:**57
fires—toxic fumes and
  gases, **6:**40–41
first aid, **5:**58, **6:**41–42
fitness. *See* physical activity
  and health

fitness and safety. *See*
  sports and injuries
fitness centers, **4:**60–61
flashback, **1:**90
flu (influenza), **8:**104–105,
  105t
food:
  addictions, **4:**61
  allergies, **4:**61–62
  irradiated, **4:**62–63, *62t*
  preparation, **4:**63–64
  safety, **6:**93–94
food-borne illnesses,
  4:134–136, **8:**131–132
food pyramids, **4:**64–66,
  65i, 121i
foreplay, **3:**55–56
foreskin, **3:**57
fracture, bone, **4:**136–137
freebasing, **1:**97
free radicals, **4:**22
fructose, **4:**118
fungal infections, **8:**85
fungi, **8:**81

G

gallstones, **8:**85–86
gang prevention efforts,
  5:59
gangs, **5:**59–60
garbage disposal, **6:**42–43
gases, **6:**43–44
gay men and women, **7:**45.
  See also homosexuality;
  same-sex relationships
gender and nutrition,
  4:66–67
generalized anxiety disorder (GAD), **2:**31–32
genes, **1:**24, **7:**50
gene therapy, **8:**86
genetically modified foods,
  4:*79f*
genetic disorders, **8:**86–87
  Down syndrome, **8:**78
  sickle-cell anemia, **8:**134
  Tay-Sachs disease,
    8:140–141
genetic engineering, **8:**87
genetics and addiction,
  1:23–24
genetic screening, **8:***87f*
genital herpes, **3:**56,
  7:45–47, 113
genital warts, **7:**47,
  113–114
gestation, **3:***94f*, 103
gestational diabetes,
  3:56–57, **4:**67
glans, **3:**57
glaucoma, **8:***84t*, 87–88

global warming, 6:44–45
glucose, 4:*118f*, 8:71
glycogen, 4:32
going steady. *See* dating; monogamy
goiter, 4:80
gonads, 3:58
gonococcal conjunctivitis, 7:47–48
gonorrhea, 3:58–59, 7:48–49. *See also* sexually transmitted diseases (STDs)
penicillin-resistant, 7:50
gout, 8:88
graffiti, 5:59
greenhouse effect, 6:45–46
grief, 2:53–54, *53f*, 114
groundwater, 6:46–47
group dating, 3:59
group therapy, 2:54–55, *54i*
growth disorders, 8:88–89
Guillain-Barre syndrome, 8:120
gun deaths, children and teens, 5:*62f*
gun laws, 5:61
gun safety, 5:61–62, *61f*
gunshot injuries, 5:62–63
guns in schools. *See* school violence
gynecologist, 3:59–60

H

HAART (highly active antiretroviral therapy), 7:23, 93
hallucinations, 1:97, 2:49, 79
hallucinogens, 1:97–99, *98t*, 2:*47t*
Hansen's disease, 8:108
Hantavirus infections (HFRS), 8:89–90
harassment, 5:63–64
hashish, 1:99
hate crimes, 5:65–66
hazardous waste disposal, 6:47–49, *48i*
asbestos, 6:*21f*
nuclear waste, 6:58–59
waste isolation pilot plant, 6:85–86
hazing, 5:66
headache, migraine, 8:118
head injuries, 5:67
health insurance, 8:90–91, *90f*
health maintenance organizations (HMO), 8:90–91

health screening, adult, 8:91, *91t*
hearing loss, 6:*58f*
heart attack, 4:45. *See also* cardiac arrest
heart defects, 8:91–92
heart disease, 1:99–100, 8:*49t*, 129–130. *See also* cardiovascular disease; coronary heart disease
heart murmur, 8:92
helmets, bike, 8:19, *77f*
helmets, use of, 5:67, *92f*
Help-911, 1:100
hemophilia, 7:50–51, 8:92
hepatitis, 1:100, 3:60–61, *61f*, 7:51–53, 8:10, 92–93, 101
herbicides, 6:49–50. *See also* insecticides
herbs and pregnancy, 3:61–64, *62–63t*
hereditary disease, 8:86–87
hermaphrodite, 3:64
heroin, 1:100–102
herpes, 3:56, 7:45–47, 53–54. *See also* sexually transmitted diseases (STDs)
heterosexuality, 3:64–65, 7:54–55
high blood pressure, 1:102–103, 4:67–68, 8:93–94, *94t*
during pregnancy, 3:65
highly active antiretroviral therapy (HAART), 7:23, 93
HIV/AIDS, 1:103, 3:65–67, 142–143, 7:62–66, *64f*. *See also* AIDS
cases by exposure category, 7:*76t*
concerns and fears, 7:110–111
confidentiality and, 7:37–38
deaths from, 7:40–42, *41f*
education about, 7:55–56
employment and, 7:56–57
health insurance and, 7:57–58, *57c*
history of, 7:58–60
infants and, 7:118–119
IV drug use and, 7:62, 115–117
by region, 7:*108t*
reporting and tracking, 7:60–61
social consequences, 7:61
STDs treatment and, 7:*95f*

teen example, 7:118–119
treatment of, 7:*58f*, 118–119, 8:*103i*
weight training and, 4:*128f*
HIV and AIDS education, 7:55–56
HIV and AIDS, employment and, 7:56–57
HIV and AIDS, health insurance and, 7:57–58, *57c*
HIV and AIDS, history of, 7:58–60
HIV and AIDS, reporting and tracking, 7:60–61
HIV and AIDS, social consequences of, 7:61
HIV and IV drug use,
HIV infections, 7:62, 115–117
HMOs (health maintenance organizations), 8:90–91
Hodgkin's disease, 8:94–95
homeopathy, 6:20, 8:26
homicide, 5:68–70, *69t*, *70f*
homicide deaths, children and teens, 5:*69f*
homophobia. *See* gay men and women; homosexuality
homosexuality, 3:148, 7:66. *See also* same-sex relationships
hormone-replacement therapy (HRT), 8:95, 116–117
hormones, 1:189, 3:67–68, 4:*114f*
hotel fires, 5:70–71
hotlines, suicide, 2:102
hot-tub drownings. *See* drowning
huffing, 1:103
Human Genome Project, 8:*87f*
human papillomavirus (HPV), 3:68–69, *69i*, 7:66–68
hunger. *See* appetite and hunger
Huntington's disease, 8:95
hydrocarbons, 6:30
hymen, 3:78
hyperbaric treatment, 5:30
hypercholesterolemia, 8:96
hypersomia, 2:90
hypertension, 8:93–94, *94t*
hyperthyroidism, 8:*142t*
hypnosis, 2:55
hypnotherapy, 1:103–104

hypothalamus, 3:70
hypothyroidism, 8:*142t*
hysterectomy, 8:96

I

illegal drugs, 1:104, 157–158. *See also* drugs
intravenous use of, 1:107
immune system, 7:68–68
immunity, 8:96–98
immunization, 8:98, *98t*
immunosuppressants, 7:69
immunotherapy, 7:69–70, 8:98–99
impetigo, 8:99
implantation, 3:37
incest, 3:70–71
incontinence, 8:156–157
infants and HIV, 7:118–119
infectious diseases, 8:99–103
number of new cases, 8:*100f*, *100t*
treatment of, 8:103–104
influenza, 8:104–105, *105t*
inhalants, 1:105
injections, 1:105
injuries, 8:105
addiction and, 1:24–25
alcohol and, 5:21–22
in America, history of, 5:72–73
back, 5:26
brain, 5:107–108
burn, 5:29–33, *31f*, *32t*
exercise and, 4:54–56
falls and, 1:54–56, 154–155
on farms, 5:*73f*
gunshot, 5:62–63
head, 5:67
inline-skating, 5:75
intentional, 5:73
motorcycle, 5:81–82
motor-vehicle, 1:153–154, 5:82–86, *83t*, *86f*
neck, 5:67
occupational, 5:73–74, *74c*
pedestrian, 5:87–88
public-transportation, 5:90
recreational and leisure, 5:92–93
repetitive-motion, 5:93–94, *94f*
roller-blade, 5:75
scooters and, 5:*93f*
skateboard, 5:100–101
spinal, 5:67

injuries (*Continued*)
  sports and. *See* sports and
    injuries
  unintentional, 5:75
  young people and,
    5:13–15, 71–72, *72f*
injuries and young people,
  5:13–15, 71-72, *72f*
injuries, intentional, 5:73
injuries, occupational,
  5:73–74, *74c*
injuries, unintentional, 5:75
insecticides, 6:50–51
insomia, 2:88
insulin, 8:71, 106
insulin-dependent diabetes.
  See diabetes mellitus
insurance, health, 8:90–91,
  90f
integrative couples therapy,
  2:*59f*
interferon, 8:106
Internet and violence,
  5:75–76
intimacy, 3:71
intimate partner violence,
  3:137–138. *See also*
  domestic violence
intoxication, 1:105–107
intramural sports, 4:68–69
intrauterine device (IUD),
  3:71–72, 7:70–71
intravenous use of illegal
  drugs, 1:107
iron, 4:69
irrational behavior, 2:55–56
irritable bowel syndrome
  (IBS), 4:60
isokinetic exercise, 4:69–70
isotonic exercise, 4:70

J

jails and violence, 5:76–77
jaundice, 7:*50f*
job-related injury, 5:73–74
jogging, 4:70–71
juvenile justice system,
  5:77–79
juveniles, 5:*59f*
juveniles and violence, 5:*78t*

K

Kaposi's sarcoma, 7:71–72,
  71i
ketamine, 1:71
kidney disorders,
  8:106–107
kissing, 3:72–73
kissing disease. *See* mononucleosis, infectious

Klinefelter's syndrome,
  8:107
knee and elbow pads. *See*
  safety equipment

L

labor, 3:73–74, *74i*
lactose, 4:*118f*
lactose intolerance, 4:*118f*
lamaze method. *See* pre-
  pared childbirth
landfills, 6:*43i*, 51–52
  Love Canal disaster,
    6:54
  waste generation rates,
    6:*82c*
laparoscopy, 3:*45f*
laryngitis, **8:107**
late term abortions, 3:*23f*
laws:
  on abortion, 3:23–24
  alcohol regulation,
    1:51–52
  antismoking, 1:59
  carbon monoxide regula-
    tion, 6:52–53
  drug, 1:87–88
  for drunk-driving, 5:51
  gun regulations, 5:61
  mental illness and,
    2:56–57, *57t*
  STD reporting, 7:72–73
  tobacco regulations,
    1:144–145, *145t*
  zero tolerance, 1:151,
    163
lead, 6:*17t, 31f*
lead poisoning, 6:53–54,
  53f
learning disabilities, **8:108**
legal interventions,
  5:79–80
Legionnaires' disease,
  8:108
legumes, 4:71
leprosy, **8:108**
lesbians, 7:73. *See also* gay
  men and women;
  same-sex relationships
leukemia, **8:109**, *109t*
life expectancy, 5:107
life support, 5:*46f*
lifetime activities, 4:71–72
life vests. *See* drowning
ligaments, 4:54–55, 102,
  139–140
liposuction, 4:145–146
liquid ecstasy, 1:71
liquor. *See* alcohol
liver disease, **8:109–110**

loud music and hearing
  damage, 6:98–99
Lou Gehrig's disease, 8:28
Love Canal, New York,
  6:54
low blood pressure, 8:110
LSD, 1:107–108
lumpectomy, 8:114
lung cancer, 1:108–110,
  109i, 8:110
  deaths among women,
    1:*141f*
  tobacco use and,
    1:156–157
lung diseases, 8:81, 111
lupus, 8:111
Lyme disease, 14, 8:101,
  111, *111f*
lymphocyte, 7:68
lymphoma, 8:94–95, 112

M

macrophage, 7:68
macular degeneration,
  8:*84t*
MADD. *See* Mothers
  Against Drunk Driving
magnetic resonance imag-
  ing (MRI), 8:118
ma huang, 8:*121f*
mainlining, 1:110
malaria, 8:112–113
male sex organs, 3:111
malignant, 1:63
malignant tumors, 8:36,
  41. *See also* cancer
malnutrition, 1:118
mammogram, 3:74–75
mammography, 8:*46i*, 113
mania, 2:57–58
marathons, 4:72–73
Marburg hemorrhagic
  fever, 8:113
marijuana, 1:99, 110–112,
  111c, 8:*22t*
marital problems, 2:58–60,
  58f
marital therapy, 2:60
marriage, 3:75–77
mastectomy, 8:113–114.
  See also breast cancer
masturbation, 3:77,
  147–148, 7:73–74
MD (muscular dystrophy),
  8:120
measles, 8:114–115
media pressures and sex,
  3:77
mediation, 2:60–61
melanoma, 8:*115t*,
  115–116

memory decline with age,
  2:40
men and nutrition. *See*
  gender and nutrition
menarche. *See* menstrual
  cycle
meningitis, 8:116
menopause, 3:78,
  8:116–117
menstrual cycle, 3:78–79
menstruation, 3:79–80
mental health, 2:61–62
  addiction and, 2:20–22,
    22c
  AIDS and, 2:23–24
  drug abuse and, 2:46–49,
    47t, 48c
  illegal drugs use and,
    1:157–158
  mental health problems,
    2:62–64
  Mental Health Parity Act,
    2:56–57
mental health professionals,
  2:*79f*
mental illness, 2:*35t, 63t,*
  64–66, *64f*, 8:117
  chances of developing,
    2:13–15
  crime and, 2:66–67
  laws and, 2:56–57, *57t*
mental retardation, 8:117
mercury, 6:*31f*, 54–55
mescaline, 1:112
metabolism, 1:52, 4:35–36
metastasis, 8:41, 117
methadone, 1:113
methamphetamine,
  1:113–115, *114c*
microbe, 7:*50f*
microbicides, 7:*87f*
microorganisms, 6:76
migraine headache, 8:118
mill tailings, 6:84
minerals, 4:73
mining:
  miners and air quality,
    6:55–56
  soil and land pollution
    from, 6:68
miscarriage, 3:80
monogamy, 3:80–81
mononucleosis, infectious,
  8:118
monounsaturated fats, 4:74
mood disorders, 2:67–68
morbidity, 5:80–81
morning after pill. *See*
  emergency contraceptive
  pills
morning sickness. *See* pregnancy, first trimester

mortality, **2:**99t, **5:**30f, **7:**40–42
mosquitoes and disease spread
  dengue fever, **8:**70
  malaria, **8:**112–113
Mothers Against Drunk Driving (MADD), **1:**82, **5:**81
motorcycle injuries, **5:**81–82
motor-vehicle injuries, **1:**153–154, **5:**82–86, 83t, 86f
movie violence, **5:**106
MRI (magnetic resonance imaging), **8:**118
multiple sclerosis (MS), **8:**118–119, 159–160
multiple-sex partners, **7:**74–75, 74t
mumps, **8:**119–120
murder. See homicide
muscle spasms, strains, and sprains, **4:**136
muscular dystrophy (MD), **8:**120
mutation, **8:**41

N

naltrexone, **1:**115
narcolepsy, **2:**90
narcotics, **1:**115–117, 116t. See also drugs
natural resources conservation, **6:**34
naturopathy, **6:**20, **8:**26
neck injuries, **5:**67
needle exchanges, **7:**75–76
negotiating sexual wants, **3:**81–82, **7:**76–77
negotiation, **5:**68f
nervous system degenerative disorders, **8:**69–70
neutrophil, **7:**68
nicotine, **1:**24, 138
nicotine replacement products, **1:**60, **117–118**
nitrates, **4:**22, 102
nitrogen oxides, **6:**17t, 19c
noise pollution, **6:**57–58, 98–99
  productivity and, **6:**57f
nomadic lifestyle, **6:**36
noncommunicable diseases, **8:**120
Nonoxynol-9, **3:**125f
nonprescription drugs, **1:**118
norepinephrine, **2:**29, 32, 41

Norplant, **3:**30–31
nuclear power plants, **6:**36, 95–96
nuclear waste, **6:**58–59, 85–86
nuclei, **6:**69f
nurse-midwife, **3:**82–83
nutrient, **4:**42
  density, **4:**74–75
nutrition:
  breast-feeding and, **4:**78–79
  cancer and, **4:**41
  drug use and, **1:**118
  health and, **4:**79–81, 80i
  labels, **4:**83–84
  pregnancy and, **3:**83–85, **4:**82
nutritional guidelines, **4:**75–76
nutritional planning, **4:**76–78
nutritional supplements, **4:**78
nutritionist, **4:**77

O

obesity, **4:**84, **8:**120–121
obesity and illness, **4:**84–88
obsessions, **2:**32, 69
obsessive-compulsive disorder (OCD), **2:**68–70, 117–118
obstetrician, **3:**85
occupational exposure guidelines, **6:**39
occupational injuries, **5:**73–74
occupational poisoning, **6:**59–60
Occupational Safety and Health Administration (OSHA), **6:**52–53, 60–61, 60f
OCD (obsessive compulsive disorder), **2:**68–70, 117–118
oil spills, **6:**35–36, 61
opiates, **1:**119
opportunistic infections, **7:**40
oral cancer, **1:**119, **8:**121, 121f
oral contraceptives, **3:**86, 92i
oral sex, **3:**86, **7:**77, 77f
organic brain disorders. See dementia
organic foods, **6:**62–63
orgasm, **3:**86–87, **7:**73

OSHA. See Occupational Safety and Health Administration **6:**60–61, 60f
osteoarthritis, **8:**31–32
osteomyelitis, **8:**121
osteoporosis, **3:**83f, **4:**88–89, **8:**121–122
ostracized, **5:**97f
otitis media, **8:**79–80
ovarian cancer, **8:**122
ovaries, **3:**87–88
overdose, alcohol, **1:**53, **5:**22–23
overdose, drug, **1:**88–89, 164–165, **5:**48–49
overdose and suicide. See suicide
overuse injury, **4:**54
overweight, **4:**89. See also obesity
ovulation, **3:**49
ovum, **3:**88
OxyContin, **1:**22f
oxytocin, **3:**90f
ozone, **6:**17t, 63–64, 99. See also air quality

P

pacemaker, **8:**122, 123i
pancreatic cancer, **8:**122–123
pancreatitis, **8:**123–124
panic attacks, **2:**32, 70
panic disorder, **2:**70–72
pap smear, **3:**88–89
pap test, **8:**124
paralysis, **5:**107
paranoia, **1:**41, **2:**21, 73, **5:**97f
paraplegia, **8:**124
paraplegic, **5:**67
parasite, **7:**23, **8:**78
parasitic infections, **8:**124
parasomia, **2:**90
Parkinson's disease, **8:**125
parole, **5:**68
partial birth abortions, **3:**23f
particulate matter, **6:**17, 17t, 19c, 64–65, 78–79
partner abuse, **5:**87
passive smoking. See secondhand smoke
pathogens, **8:**99f
PCBs (polychlorinated biphenyls), **6:**69
PCP, **1:**120
pedestrian injuries, **5:**87–88
peer pressure, **4:**89–90, **5:**38f
  addiction and, **1:**121
  drug use and, **1:**170–171

sexual behaviors and, **3:**135–136
peer relationships and mental health, **1:**170–171. See also social support systems
peer relationships and sexuality, **7:**77–78
pellagra, **4:**121
pelvic inflammatory disease (PID), **7:**78
penicillin, **8:**125
penis, **3:**89, 89f
pentamidine, **7:**78–79
perinatal period, **3:**89–91
perineum, **3:**49
period. See menstruation
peritonitis, **8:**30–31
personality, **2:**72
personality disorders, **2:**72–74, 73t
personal trainer, **4:**91
pertussis, **8:**148
pesticides, **6:**30–31, 65–66, 99–100. See also herbicides
phobias, **2:**74–76, 75t
pH scale, **6:**15i
physical activity and health, **4:**91–94, 91f
  aging and, **4:**92f
  guidelines for, **4:**95
  inactivity and related diseases, **4:**98–101
  mental health and, **4:**94
  pyramid, **4:**93i
  safety of, **4:**146–148
physical education class, **4:**98f, 100–101t
physical fitness, **4:**13–15
  planning, **4:**95–98, 97t
phytochemicals, **4:**22
PID (pelvic inflammatory disease), **7:**78
pill, the. See oral contraceptives
pitchblende, **6:**84
placenta, **3:**91
plague, bubonic, **8:**125–126
plan B. See emergency contraceptive pills
Planned Parenthood, **3:**91–93, 92f, 142
plateau, **4:**109
pleurisy, **8:**126
pneumonia, **7:**79, **8:**108, 126–127
poisoning
  drug and alcohol, **1:**53–54, **5:**88–89
  first aid for, **6:**41–42
  risks of, **6:**11–13

poliomyelitis, 8:127

pollutant standards index (PSI), 6:66–67, 66c

pollution
  agricultural, 6:67–68
  air, 6:16–17, 17t, 29i
  chemical, 6:29–32
  noise, 6:57–58, 57f, 98–99
  non-point source, 6:34, 87
  point source, 6:85, 87
  soil and land, 6:68–69
  thermal, 6:79–80
  water, 6:87–88, 91–92

polychlorinated biphenyls (PCBs), 6:69

polygamy, 3:93

pornography, 3:93

postpartum blues, 2:76f, 3:93

postpartum depression, 2:76–77, 76f, 3:94

posttraumatic-stress disorder (PTSD), 2:77, 112–113

preeclampsia, 3:65

pregnancy, 3:94–97, 95f, 96c
  exercise, 3:49–50, 50f, 4:56
  first trimester, 3:97–98
  herbs and, 3:61–64, 62–63t
  high blood pressure during, 3:65
  HIV transmission during, 8:23
  prevention of, 3:20, 30, 47, 51f, 98–102, 101t, 142
  risks of, 3:145
  second trimester, 3:102–103, 103i
  third trimester, 3:103–104
  tobacco, alcohol, and drug use and, 1:122–123, 122c, 3:24–25
  unintended. See unintended pregnancy
  weight and, 4:101–102

premature labor, 3:43

prenatal care, 3:104–105, 4:101–102

prenatal development, 3:105–107

prenuptial agreement, 3:75f

prepared childbirth, 3:107–108

prescription drugs:
  addiction and, 1:21–23, 158
  drug overdose and, 1:164–165
  illegal use of, 1:171

preservatives in foods, 4:102–103

prisons. See jails

probation, 5:89

processed foods, 4:103–104

productivity and noise pollution, 6:57

product recalls, 5:95f

progestins, 3:108

prophylaxis, 7:79

prostate cancer, 8:127–128

protective clothing. See safety equipment

proteins, 4:104–105

psychiatrist, 2:79

psychoactive, 1:120f

psychoactive drugs, 1:123–124

psychologist, 2:79

psychosis, 1:124, 2:79–80

psychotherapy, 2:80–82, 81f

PTSD (posttraumatic-stress disorder), 2:77, 112–113

puberty, 3:108–109, 145–146

public-transportation injuries, 5:90

pulmonary disease, chronic obstructive (COPD), 8:60, 60t

pulse, 4:105

purging, 4:38

pyramids, food, 4:64–66, 65i, 121i

Q

quackery, 8:128. See also alternative medicine

R

R.I.C.E., 4:54

rabies, 8:128–129

radiation, 6:58–59, 69–70, 69f

radiation therapy, 8:47–48

radioactive processed foods. See food, irradiated

radon gas, 6:13, 44, 71–72, 92

range of motion. See exercise, flexibility and

rape, 3:125–126, 5:90–91. See also sexual assault and rape

rape crisis centers, 5:91–92

raves, 1:124–125

RDA for pregnant women, 3:84t

recalls of products, 5:95f

recreational and leisure injuries, 5:92–93

recycling, 6:72–74
  conservation and, 6:34, 100
  process of, 6:73–74, 74i
  rates by product, 6:73c
  uses for products, 6:72–73

relapse, 1:20

relaxation therapy, 2:82–85

repetitive-motion injuries, 5:93–94, 94f

reporting and tracking HIV/AIDS, 7:60–61

reporting and tracking STDs, 7:72–73, 92–93

repression, 2:39

reproductive organs:
  female, 3:110–111
  male, 3:111

reproductive technologies, 3:112

resistance, 7:50

respiratory diseases and tobacco use, 1:141–142

resuscitation, 3:43f

retinal detachment, 8:84t

retrovirus, 7:80

ReVia, 1:115

Reye's syndrome, 8:129

rheumatic heart disease, 8:129–130

rheumatoid arthritis, 8:31–32

Rh factor, 3:104f

rhythm method, 3:112

rickets, 4:80

Ritalin, 2:33f

road rage, 5:94

Rocky Mountain spotted fever, 8:130

Roe v. Wade. See abortion, laws concerning

Rohypnol, 1:71

roller-blade injuries, 5:75

RU-486. See abortion

rubella, 8:130

running. See jogging

rush, 1:41, 113

S

SAD. See seasonal affective disorder

Safe Drinking Water Act, 6:46–47, 86, 88

safe houses, 5:68f

safer sex, 3:112–113, 7:80–82

safety belts, 5:94–95, 94f

safety equipment, 5:95, 95f

safety rules, general, 5:95–96

Salmonella, 8:131–132

same-sex relationships, 3:113–115, 148. See also homosexuality

sarcoma, 8:132

satiety, 4:34

saturated fats, 4:106

scabies, 7:82

scarlet fever, 8:132

schizophrenia, 2:85–87, 85f, 86i, 111–112

school sports, 4:106–107

school violence, 5:80f, 96–99, 98t. See also violence, mental health and

scoliosis, 8:132

scooters and injuries, 5:93f

screening, genetic, 8:87f

screening, health, adult, 8:91, 91t

scurvy, 4:107

seasonal affective disorder (SAD), 2:87, 113–114

seat belts, 5:94–95, 94f

secondhand smoke, 1:125, 141

self-help groups, 5:42, 101. See also support groups

self-injury, 2:123

semen, 3:115

septic systems, 6:74–75

serotonin, 2:29, 32, 41

serving size, 4:107–108, 108t

set point, 4:108–109

sewage, 6:75–76

sex. See sexual intercourse

sex, alcohol, and drugs, 1:41–42, 3:115–116, 115f, 7:25–26

sex during and after pregnancy, 3:116–117

sex organs:
  female, 3:110–111
  male, 3:111

sexual abuse. See dating abuse; incest; sexual assault and rape

sexual activity, 7:82–83, *83c. See also* sexual intercourse
sexual assault and rape, **3:117–120**, *117f, 119c, 120f*, **125–126**, 137, **5:90–91**, 99
sexual characteristics, 3:120
sexual harassment, **5:100**
sexual intercourse, 3:27–28, 120, 7:27–28. *See also* contraception; sexual activity; unintended pregnancy
sexuality, 3:121–122
sexually transmitted diseases (STDs), **3:122–123**, 7:12–16, 84–87, *96t*, 8:133
  confidentiality and, 7:37–38
  deaths from, 7:40–42
  diagnosing, 7:91
  drugs and, 7:89–90
  history of, 7:91–92
  laws about reporting, 7:72–73
  pregnancy and, 7:90, *90t*
  reporting and tracking, 7:92
  risk of infection, 3:144–145
  risky behaviors, 3:16–18
  teens and, 7:101–103
  testing for, 7:96–97
  treatment for, 3:136–137, **7:92–96**
sexual orientation. *See* bisexuality; gay men and women; heterosexuality; homosexuality; lesbian
sex workers, 7:87–88
shelters, domestic violence, 5:44
shingles, 7:88–89, 8:133–134
shoplifting and mental health, 2:121–122
sick building syndrome (SBS), 6:76–77
sickle-cell anemia, 8:134
side-stream smoke. *See* secondhand smoke
sigmoidoscopy, 8:39
sinusitis, 8:134
skateboard injuries, 5:100–101
skeletal muscles, 4:109–110
skin cancer, 4:110–111, 8:115–116, *115t*, 134–135

skin disorders, 8:135–136
sleep apnea, 2:90
sleep disorders, 2:88–90, *88f*, 8:136–137
sleep requirements, 8:*136t*
sludge, 6:47
smallpox, 8:137
smog, 6:77–78
smoke detectors, 5:101
smokeless tobacco, 1:127–128
smokestack scrubbers, 6:78–79
smoking. *See also* tobacco; tobacco use
  addiction risk, 1:166–167
  antismoking laws, 1:59, *126–127t*
  antismoking products, 1:59–61
  deaths from, 1:*137f*
  depression and, 5:*105f*
  fires and, 5:101
  health risks from, 6:12, 80–81, 98, 8:9–10, 19, *111f*
  pregnancy and, 3:123–125, *124c, 124f*
  weight gain when quitting, 1:168–169
smoking cessation, 1:128–130, 167–169
sobriety checkpoints, 5:49
social consequences of weight, 4:112–113
social norms, 5:38
social phobia, 2:109–110
social pressures, 5:59. *See also* peer pressure
social support systems, 2:91
socioeconomic status, 5:42
sodium, 4:113
soil and land pollution, 6:68–69
somatoform disorders, 2:91–92
spasms, muscle, 4:136
speculum, 3:20
speech disorders. *See* mental retardation
sperm, 3:125
spermicides, 3:125, 7:89
SPF (sun protection factor), 4:*53f*
spinal injuries, 5:67
sports and injuries, 4:113–114, 139–140, 147–148, 5:92–93
sports and nutrition, 4:114
spousal abuse, 5:101–102. *See also* domestic violence

sprains, muscle, 4:136
stalking, 5:*42f*
starch, 4:32, 42
statutory rape, 3:125–126
STDs. *See* sexually transmitted diseases
  STDs and drugs, 7:89–90
  STDs and pregnancy, 7:90, *90t*
  STDs, diagnosing, 7:91
  STDs, history of, 7:92
  STDs, reporting and tracking, 7:92
  STDs, treatment of, 3:136–137, 7:92–96
  STD testing, 7:96–97
stenosis, 8:137
sterile, 6:30
steroids, anabolic, 1:58
steroids and weight gain, 4:114–116, *116f*
stillbirth, 3:43
stimulants, 1:130–131, *130t*, 2:*47t*
stop, drop, and roll, 5:102
strains, muscle, 4:136
strength exercises, 4:116–117
strep throat, 8:137–138
stress, 2:93–96, *93f, 94t*, 8:138–139
  chronic, 2:110–111
  immune system and, 2:96–97
  management techniques, 2:82–85, 8:138–139
stressors, 2:110–111
stretching exercises, 4:117
stroke, 8:139, *139t*
substance abuse, 1:20
sucrose, 4:118
sugar, 4:118
suicide, 2:98–102, 5:102–105, *104t*
  attempts, 2:102, 118, 5:105
  cost of, 2:*100f*
  death rates, 2:*99t*
  demographics, 2:*99f*
  depression and, 8:*70f*
  by firearms, 2:124
  grieving after, 2:114
  helping someone, 2:*101f-102f*
  hotlines, 2:102
  prevalence among homosexuals, 2:120–121
  warning signs, 2:103
sulfites, 4:22, 102
sulfur dioxide, 6:*17t*, 19, *19c*, 78, 93

sun protection factor (SPF), 4:*53f*
Superfund, 6:79
supplements, dietary, 8:*121f*
support groups, 1:131–132, 2:103–104, 8:139
  Al-Anon, 1:30–31
  Alateen, 1:31
  Alcoholics Anonymous, 1:48
  for pregnant teens, 3:134–135
  twelve-step programs, 1:148–149
Surgeon General's warnings, 1:132
surgery, 8:47–48, 50, 58–59
swimming, 4:118–119
syphilis, 3:126–127, 7:98–99, *99t*, 8:139–140
systemic infections, 8:140
systemic lupus erythematosus, 8:111
systolic pressure, 8:140

T
tai chi, 4:119
tanning machines, 8:166
tar. *See* tobacco, chemicals in
Tay-Sachs disease, 8:140–141
T-cells, 7:99–100
teen pregnancy, 3:*95f, 96c*, 127–128, *127f-128f*
teens and addiction, 1:*134c*, 135–136, *136t*
teens and AIDS, 7:100–101, *100t*
teens and sexually transmitted diseases, 7:101–103
television violence, 5:106
tendon, 4:109
teratogens, 1:90, 141, 3:*94f*
testes, 3:128
testicular cancer, 8:141
testosterone, 3:128–129
tetanus, 8:141
thermal pollution, 6:79–80
Three Mile Island nuclear power plant, 6:36
throat cancer, 1:136
thyroid disorders, 8:141–142, *142t*
tic disorders, 2:105–106
tinnitus, 6:57

tobacco, **1:136–137**. *See also* smoking; tobacco use
addiction, **1:137–140**
chemicals in, **1:142–143**
forms of, **1:143–144,** *143f*
laws regulating, **1:144–145,** *145t*
settlements, **1:146–148,** *146t-147t*
smoke from, **6:***31f,* **80–81**
tobacco, chemicals in, **1:142–143**
tobacco, forms of, **1:143–144,** *143f*
tobacco use. *See also* smoking; tobacco
advertising and media, **1:28–30**
clean air policies in U.S., **1:***126–127t*
depression and, **2:122–123**
health problems from, **1:16–18, 140–141**
lung cancer and, **1:156–157**
pregnancy and, **1:122–123,** *122c*
respiratory diseases, **1:141–142**
secondhand smoke, **1:125**
victims of, **1:***138f,* *140f*
tolerance, **1:20, 49, 148, 2:21**
Tourette's disorder. *See* tic disorders
toxic chemicals, **6:***31f,* **40–41, 81, 96–97**
toxic cleanup. *See* Superfund
toxic shock syndrome, **3:129–130, 8:143**
transcendental mediation, **2:60–61**
transfusion, **7:***30f*
transplants:
  bone marrow, **8:35–36**
  donor cards, **8:78**

transuranic waste, **6:85**
trash, **6:81–83**
  burning of, **6:83**
  toxic fumes and gases from fires, **6:40–41**
  waste generation rates, **6:***82c*
trauma centers, **5:107**
traumatic brain injury, **5:107–108**
tremors, **2:23**
triathlon, **4:119–120**
trichomoniasis, **3:130, 7:103–104**
tubal ligation, **3:130–131**
tuberculosis, **8:143**
tumors, **8:36, 41, 143**
Tuskegee study, **7:104**
twelve-step program, **1:148–149,** *149–150t*
twins, **3:***37f*
Type II diabetes, **8:72, 74**
typhoid fever, **8:143–144**
typhus, **8:144**

U

ulcers, **8:144**
ultraviolet rays (UV), **6:32, 49, 63, 70, 83–84**
unintended pregnancy, **3:131**. *See also* contraception; pregnancy
  choices and actions, **3:7–8**
  risky vs. safe behaviors, **3:13–15**
  support groups, **3:134–135**
  teen fathers, **3:140–142**
  teen mothers, **3:139–140**
unintended sex. *See* sexual activity
unipolar disorders, **2:67–68**
unprotected sex, **3:131–132, 7:105,** *105f,* **112–113**
uranium mining, **6:56, 71, 84–85**
urethra, **3:57**
uterine cancer, **8:145**
uterine lining, **3:20**
uterus, **3:132**

V

vaccines, **8:***98t,* **145–146**
vagina, **3:132–133**
vaginal sex, **7:105–106**
vaginal warts, **7:106**
vaginitis, **7:106–107**
vasectomy, **3:133**
vasocongestion, **3:133**
vegetarians, **4:120,** *121i,* **144**
video game violence, **5:108**
video violence, **5:106**
violence:
  domestic/family, **1:77, 5:41–44,** *43f*
  Internet and, **5:75–76,** *75–76*
  intimate partner, **3:137–138**
  jails and, **5:76–77**
  juveniles and, **5:***78t*
  mental health and, **2:106–107**
  movie, **5:106**
  school, **5:***80f,* **96–99,** *98t*
  television, **5:106**
  video, **5:106**
  video game, **5:108**
  young people and, **5:16–18**
violence and mental health, **2:106–107**
viral infections, **8:145–146**
virginity, **7:107**
viruses, **7:23, 30, 8:25, 147**
vitamins, **4:120–122**
volatile organic compounds, **6:16,** *19c*
vomiting, **4:122–123**

W

walking and diet, **4:123**
warm-up exercises, **4:123–124**
warts. *See* human papillomavirus

waste isolation pilot plant (WIPP), **6:85–86**
water, **4:124–125**
water pollution, **6:87–88, 91–92**
watersheds, **6:89–90**
weight:
  gain when quitting smoking, **1:168–169**
  losing, **4:134, 8:***121f*
  management techniques, **4:126–128,** *127t*
  social consequences of, **4:112–113**
  weight-loss programs, **4:125–126**
weight training, **4:128–130,** *130t*
West Nile disease, **8:147–148**
white blood cells, **8:***97i*
whooping cough, **8:148**
wine. *See* alcohol
WIPP (waste isolation pilot plant), **6:85–86**
withdrawal, **1:150**
women and nutrition. *See* gender and nutrition
World Health Organization (WHO), **7:107–109**

X

xenophobia, **2:107**

Y

years of potential life lost (YPLL), **109**
yellow fever, **8:148–149**
yoga, **4:131**

Z

zero tolerance laws, **1:151, 163**
zoophobia, **2:108**
zyban, **1:151**
zygote, **3:37**